Managing Schizophrenia

Ann Mortimer
Department of Psychiatry
University of Hull School of Medicine
Hull, UK

Sean Spence
Academic Department of Psychiatry
University of Sheffield
Sheffield, UK

Published by Science Press Ltd, 34–42 Cleveland Street, London W1T 4LB, UK

© 2001 Science Press Ltd

http://www.current-science-group.com/

All rights reserved. No part of this publication may be reproduced, stored in a retrieval system or transmitted in any form or by any means electronic, mechanical, photocopying, recording or otherwise without prior written permission of the publishers.

British Library Cataloguing in Publication Data

A catalogue record for this book is available from the British Library.

ISBN 1-85873-931-4

Although every effort has been made to ensure that drug doses and other information are presented accurately in this publication, the ultimate responsibility rests with the prescribing physician. Neither the publishers nor the authors can be held responsible for errors or for any consequences arising from the use of information contained herein. Any product mentioned in this publication should be used in accordance with the prescribing information prepared by the manufacturers. No claims or endorsements are made for any drug or compound at present under clinical investigation.

Project editor: Clare Wheatcroft
Illustrator: Matthew McCutcheon
Typesettter: Ros Dignon
Designer: Simon Banister
Production: David Forrest

Printed in Italy by Offset Print Veneta S.r.l

Cover illustration: Brain regions activated by word generation.

Contents

	Biographies	v
	Acknowledgements	vi
1.	**Introduction**	**1**
	References	3
2.	**The syndromes of schizophrenia**	**4**
	The positive syndrome	4
	The negative syndrome	5
	References	8
3.	**Clinical validity of the negative syndrome**	**9**
	Prevalence	9
	Relationship of the negative syndrome to affective disorder	13
	Relationship of negative symptoms to drug treatment	13
	References	14
4.	**Neuroscience and the negative syndrome**	**17**
	Neuroimaging: structural	17
	Neuroimaging: functional	18
	Neuroimaging: spectroscopy	22
	Neurochemistry	25
	Neuropsychology	30
	Neurophysiology	31
	Conclusions	32
	References	32
5.	**The burden of negative symptoms**	**38**
	Impact on the individual and their family	38
	Economic burden	39
	References	40
6.	**Assessment of negative symptoms**	**41**
	Primary and pseudonegative symptoms	41
	Presence and severity: clinical assessment versus rating scale assessment	41
	Appraisal of clinical trial results	42
	Differential diagnoses and their management	43
	References	46
7.	**Pharmacological treatment approaches**	**47**
	General philosophy	47
	Differentiation between direct and indirect effects of neuroleptic drugs on negative symptoms	47
	Atypical neuroleptic drugs and negative symptoms	48
	Other psychotropic drugs and negative symptoms	53
	Psychotropic and other drugs ineffective against negative symptoms	55
	References	57

8.	**Social and family approaches**	**60**
	Psychosocial interventions	60
	Rehabilitation	61
	Social skills training	62
	References	63
9.	**Coordinating the delivery of services**	**64**
	Primary and secondary care	64
	Care programming approach	66
	The supervision register	66
	The general practitioner	67
	References	70
	Source material	**71**
	Further reading	**72**
	Appendices I–VII	**73**

Biographies

Professor Ann M Mortimer is Foundation Chair in Psychiatry at the University of Hull, Hull, UK. She qualified in medicine from Leicester University, Leicester, UK, where she also completed a degree in biochemistry and genetics research. She trained in psychiatry in Yorkshire, UK, including a lectureship at the University of Leeds, where she developed a research interest in schizophrenia. Following an initial consultant post in Yorkshire, she became a senior lecturer at Imperial College, London, before being appointed to her chair in 1995. Professor Mortimer has built up a substantial volume of ongoing schizophrenia research in her department, including investigations of new antipsychotic drugs, cognitive neuropsychological work and early intervention appraisal. She has additional clinical and research interests in mother and baby mental health and is currently leading curriculum development for mental health and disorder in the new Hull and York School of Medicine. Professor Mortimer has three small children.

Dr Sean A Spence is Clinical Senior Lecturer in the Academic Department of Psychiatry, University of Sheffield, Sheffield, UK. He qualified in medicine from Guy's Hospital, London, UK, where he also completed a degree in psychology. Following a period of general medical training and working in general practice he trained in psychiatry at Charing Cross and other hospitals in west London. He was a Medical Research Council (MRC) Clinical Training Fellow on the MRC Cyclotron Unit at the Hammersmith Hospital, London and subsequently a DeWitt–Wallace visiting research fellow to the functional neuroimaging laboratory of Cornell Medical Center, New York, USA. His research interests are in the field of brain imaging of the higher cognitive functions in humans in the healthy and diseased states. In 1997 he won the research prize and medal of the Royal College of Psychiatrists (London) and also the research essay prize of the Royal Society of Medicine (London). His clinical interests are in the field of schizophrenia and the psychoses and also the treatment of the homeless.

Acknowledgements

Figure 4.2. Reproduced with permission from Rajkowska G, Goldman-Rakic PS. **Cytoarchitectonic definition of prefrontal areas in normal human cortex: II. Variability in locations of areas 9 and 46 and relationship to the Talairach Coordinate System.** *Cereb Cortex* 1995; **5**:323–337.

Figure 4.3. Reproduced with permission from Liddle PF, Friston KJ, Frith CD. **Patterns of cerebral blood flow in schizophrenia.** *Br J Psychiatry* 1992; **160**:179–186.

Figure 4.4. Reproduced with permission from Chua SE, Wright IC, Poline JB *et al.* **Grey matter correlates of syndromes in schizophrenia. A semi-automated analysis of structural magnetic resonance images.** *Br J Psychiatry* 1997; **170**:406–410.

Figure 4.5. Data from Dolan RJ, Bench CJ, Liddle PF *et al.* **Dorsolateral prefrontal cortex dysfunction in the major psychoses; symptom or disease specificity?** *J Neurol Neurosurg Psychiatry* 1993; **56**:1290–1294.

Figure 4.6. Reproduced with permission from Spence SA, Hirsch SR, Brooks DJ *et al.* **Prefrontal cortex activity in people with schizophrenia and control subjects. Evidence of positron emission tomography for remission of 'hypofrontality' with recovery from acute schizophrenia.** *Br J Psychiatry* 1998; **172**:316–323.

Figure 4.7. Data from Spence SA, Liddle PF, Stefan MD *et al.* **Functional anatomy of verbal fluency in people with schizophrenia and those at genetic risk. Focal dysfunction and distributed disconnectivity reappraised.** *Br J Psychiatry* 2000; **176**:52–60.

Chapter 1

Introduction

The concept of positive versus negative symptoms did not originate within psychiatry. It was a physician, Reynolds, who in 1857 proposed that neurological symptoms could be classified as either an 'excess of vital properties' or a 'negation of vital properties' [1]. The neurologist Hughlings Jackson is credited with the application of this concept to the symptoms of mental disorder, although its original meaning has undergone modification [2]. Bleueler [3] and Kraepelin [4] both went on to define schizophrenic illness within a similar framework, in terms of 'florid' or 'accessory' symptoms (corresponding to 'positive' symptoms) coupled with 'deterioration' or 'fundamental' symptoms (which would now be recognised as 'negative'). Despite some variations in this concept, schizophrenia continued to be perceived as a composite of separate classes of symptom, even though these classes frequently coexisted in the same patient. As the 20th century progressed, these classes were described in more detail [5–7]. Eventually the modern definitions of positive and negative symptoms of schizophrenia evolved [8], together with the realisation that this distinction had wide implications for the aetiology, treatment and prognosis of the disorder [9]. In particular, positive symptoms were proposed to arise from a potentially reversible excess of dopaminergic neurotransmission in the brain, while negative symptoms were the manifestation of an irreversible degenerative process.

The validity of positive and negative syndromes has repeatedly been demonstrated by factor analytic studies. These studies infer that, statistically, groups of symptoms considered negative or positive are more closely associated with each other than with symptoms of the other class, both cross-sectionally [10–14] and longitudinally [15,16], in groups of patients ranging from 'first episode' to chronic, hospitalized samples. The association of positive symptoms with each other does not appear to be as strong as that of negative symptoms with each other; factor analytic studies have generally found positive symptoms to be divided across at least two subfactors rather than clustering altogether. The predominant view is that the subfactors of positive symptoms with most validity are: a factor consisting of thought disorder and inappropriate affect, termed the 'disorganization' syndrome and a factor consisting of delusions and hallucinations, termed the 'reality distortion syndrome' [17]. Taken together, the negative syndrome plus the above two positive sub-syndromes correspond quite well to three of the four classic clinical subtypes of schizophrenia: 'simple schizophrenia' is characterized by the negative syndrome, 'hebephrenic schizophrenia' by the disorganization syndrome and 'paranoid schizophrenia' by the reality distortion syndrome.

Despite the supposedly poor response of negative symptoms to treatment, the landmark study of Wing and Brown [8] demonstrated that reducing the social impoverishment of patients was associated with a concomitant reduction of negative symptoms. Subsequently, it has become clear that not all apparent negative symptoms are authentic. They may be mimicked by other psychopathologies such as untreated positive symptoms. As a result, the terminology applied to negative symptomatology has become increasingly complicated. The use of the term 'secondary negative symptoms' to describe aetiologically unrelated presentations, which nevertheless mimic genuine negative symptoms, has supplied particular potential for confusion. Here, the 'primary negative symptoms' are held to be authentic or 'true' negative symptoms.

Research over the last two decades has gone a long way towards generating an understanding of the essential nature of negative symptoms, together with some characterization of their pathophysiology. As is often the case with mental disorder, many experimental hypotheses have arisen from the results of attempts at drug treatment, rather than an *a priori* sound knowledge of specific aetiology informing those therapeutic interventions. Until a few years ago, accepted wisdom remained that negative symptoms were both unresponsive to neuroleptic treatment and prognostically unfavourable. The experience of most psychiatrists was that escalating residual symptoms were an inevitable accompaniment to repeated relapse and chronicity of the disorder; it seemed that there would always be a 'rump' of the worst affected patients, unable to benefit from rehabilitative efforts. These patients would remain severely disabled and unlikely to function with any degree of independence.

The introduction of atypical antipsychotic drugs has afforded at least the possibility of better management of negative symptoms. These drugs combine a reduced side effect profile with (possibly) a superior antipsychotic efficacy (in some cases pertaining to negative as well as positive symptoms). Patients who are able to respond tend to become more accessible to rehabilitation strategies, which may reduce the negative syndrome further in that its secondary disabilities and handicaps may be attenuated. It is now possible to measure and monitor negative symptoms using dedicated rating scales (eg, Schedule for the Assessment of Negative Symptoms [SANS], *see* Chapter 6), which introduce a degree of objectivity into the process. It has also been recognised that most differential diagnoses of the negative syndrome can be treated relatively effectively. Given this range of new treatment approaches, the therapeutic gloom that surrounded negative symptoms is much less justifiable than it used to be.

This book aims to provide a comprehensive 'state of the art' exposition of both the theoretical background to, and the neuroscientific underpinning of, the negative syndrome. From this theoretical underpinning, implications have been drawn for the clinical management of patients with schizophrenia and their families, which may feed into and improve upon structures and strategies currently available. It is hoped that this distillation of new knowledge from research, clinical advances and psychopharmacology into a practical guide will help those involved in patient care to recognise, diagnose and successfully treat the negative symptoms of schizophrenia.

References

1. Berrios GE. **Positive and negative symptoms and Jackson. A conceptual history.** *Arch Gen Psychiatry* 1985; **42**:95–97.
2. McKenna PJ. *Schizophrenia and Related Syndromes.* Oxford: Oxford University Press, 1994.
3. Bleueler E. *Dementia Praecox or the Group of Schizophrenias.* New York: International Universities Press, 1911.
4. Kraepelin E. *Dementia Praecox and Paraphrenia.* Edinburgh: Livingstone, 1913.
5. Schneider K. *Clinical Psychopathology. 5th edition.* New York: Grune and Stratton, 1958.
6. Jilek WG. **The residual dimension. A study of residual symptoms in veterans with chronic psychiatric illness. I.** *Psychiatr Clin (Basel)* 1968; **1**:175–191.
7. Jilek WG. **The residual dimension. A study of residual symptoms in veterans with chronic psychiatric illness. II.** *Psychiatr Clin (Basel)* 1968; **1**:193–218.
8. Wing JK, Brown GW. *Institutionalism and Schizophrenia: a Comparative Study of Three Mental Hospitals, 1960–1968.* Cambridge: Cambridge University Press, 1970.
9. Crow TJ. **Molecular pathology of schizophrenia: more than one disease process?** *Br Med J* 1980; **280**:66–68.
10. Andreasen NC, Olsen S. **Negative v positive schizophrenia. Definition and validation.** *Arch Gen Psychiatry* 1982; **39**:784–788.
11. Kulhara P, Kota SK, Joseph S. **Positive and negative subtypes of schizophrenia. A study from India.** *Acta Psychiatr Scand* 1986; **74**:353–359.
12. Mortimer AM, Lund CE, McKenna PJ et al. **Rating of negative symptoms using the High Royds Evaluation of Negativity (HEN) scale.** *Br J Psychiatry Suppl* 1989; **160**:89–92.
13. Palacios-Araus L, Herran A, Sandoya M et al. **Analysis of positive and negative symptoms in schizophrenia. A study from a population of long-term outpatients.** *Acta Psychiatr Scand* 1995; **92**:178–182.
14. Vazquez-Barquero JL, Lastra I, Cuesta Nunez MJ et al. **Patterns of positive and negative symptoms in first episode schizophrenia.** *Br J Psychiatry* 1996; **168**:693–701.
15. Rey ER, Bailer J, Brauer W et al. **Stability trends and longitudinal correlations of negative and positive syndromes within a three-year follow-up of initially hospitalized schizophrenics.** *Acta Psychiatr Scand* 1994; **90**:405–412.
16. Eaton WW, Thara R, Federman B et al. **Structure and course of positive and negative symptoms in schizophrenia.** *Arch Gen Psychiatry* 1995; **52**:127–134.
17. Liddle PF. **The syndromes of chronic schizophrenia. A re-examination of the positive-negative dichotomy.** *Br J Psychiatry* 1987; **151**:145–151.

Chapter 2

The syndromes of schizophrenia

People with schizophrenia suffer from a very broad spectrum of symptoms. Research has shown that certain clusters of symptoms more frequently associate with each other than with symptoms outside those clusters, in other words, that these groups of symptoms constitute syndromes. The positive syndrome comprises phenomena that augment the events experienced in 'normal' mental life, such as delusions and hallucinations, while the negative syndrome comprises deficits in normal mental functions, such as emotional response and motivation. The positive syndrome can be divided, on factor analytic evidence (see above), into 'reality distortion' (delusions and hallucinations) and 'disorganization' (thought disorder and inappropriate affect).

The syndromes, however, are not equivalent to patients; although the clinical state of some patients may be dominated by one syndrome, most patients will manifest symptoms from more than one syndrome at the same time during the course of their illness. For example, the balance of syndromes may differ when a patient is in acute relapse from when that same patient is stable.

The positive syndrome

Reality distortion

General medical symptoms (eg, pain, breathlessness and depression) can be envisaged by and indeed, may have been experienced by, most people. Reality distortion symptoms are unusual in this respect and are so bizarre and alien that it is difficult to imagine what it is like to suffer from them. Overall, reality distortion can be interpreted as a loss of boundary of the self, not knowing where the self ends and the rest of the world begins. Reality distortion symptoms fall into this category, and are of great diagnostic importance, although they do not predict outcome. They are generally considered to respond fairly well to neuroleptic treatment in most patients.

Reality distortion symptoms of schizophrenia include the following.
- Delusions: bizarre false beliefs, which may be persecutory, grandiose or indicative of false memories.
- Hallucinations: false perceptions without real origin (classically these are voices, but they can be in any sensory modality).
- Passivity: feeling controlled or influenced in action, thought or affect by an outside force.
- Interference with thinking: thoughts are not one's own (thought insertion), are stolen (thought withdrawal) or are broadcast and picked up by others.
- Delusional mood: a pervasive belief that something of momentous import is about to happen.

- Delusions of reference: attributing abnormal significance to ordinary surroundings or events, or to the expressions of other people.

The above symptoms are usually accompanied by an affect of fear, suspicion or apprehension that is quite understandable. Many patients become withdrawn and guarded and will not admit to their abnormal beliefs and experiences. Objective evidence of reality distortion and possibly other 'positive' symptoms may be observed. The symptoms may manifest in the following ways.

- Hallucinatory behaviour: conversing with or gesticulating towards voices/visions, mumbling to self.
- Arranging objects or dressing in a 'special' way: peculiar rituals.
- Disinhibited social or sexual behaviours.
- Abnormal motor behaviours such as mannerisms and stereotypies (purposeless, repetitive behaviours).
- Outbursts of verbal or physical aggression.

Disorganization

The disorganization syndrome accounts for much less variance than the reality distortion and negative syndromes in factor analytic studies. The disorganization syndrome is now considered to be unrelated to the negative syndrome. Disorganization may not be necessary for a diagnosis of schizophrenia, but, if present, is thought to imply a poor prognosis. Its response to neuroleptic treatment is variable. Unlike reality distortion symptoms, the symptoms of disorganization are in the main observed by others rather than complained of by the patient.

The disorganization symptoms include the following.

- Thought disorder: derailment, tangentiality, illogicality and incoherence. Thought disorder results in fluent speech that is compromised in its ability to convey meaning to the listener. It ranges from pedantic 'officialese' to an unintelligible 'word salad', where sentence structure breaks down and new words (neologisms) may appear.
- Inappropriate affect: incongruous smiling, giggling or laughter in short bursts for no apparent reason. In severe form, the patient appears chronically fatuous and disinhibited.

The negative syndrome

The negative syndrome implies an inability to respond to stimuli, whether these are internally or externally generated. Thus, there is a lack (a 'poverty') of normal mental activity and its consequences. This is most noticeable in ideation (thought) and emotional response. It seems likely that the other hallmarks of the negative syndrome, such as poor social function (see below) are secondary to these basic deficits. Unfortunately, the term 'secondary negative symptoms' has been used to describe similar, but unrelated, presentations such as depression and Parkinsonism in patients with schizophrenia; these may mimic the negative syndrome to the untrained observer. The authors suggest the term 'pseudonegative symptoms' to describe these presentations (*see* Table 2.1).

Classification of negative symptoms		
Symptom type	Cause	Result
Primary	Pathophysiology of schizophrenia: failure to respond	Poverty of ideation Poverty of affect
	Consequences of primary symptoms	Loss of motivation Poverty of speech Poverty of behaviour Loss of self-care
Pseudonegative	Parkinsonism Unresolved positive symptoms Depression Oversedation Institutional environment Schizoid premorbid personality	Any of the above, plus additional symptoms specific to the cause of pseudonegative symptoms

Table 2.1

To complicate matters further, negative symptoms have also been classified according to whether they have been assessed cross-sectionally or whether they have been shown to persist over time [1]. Thus, plain 'negative symptoms' might refer to primary or pseudo, temporary or permanent symptoms. Primary symptoms that are also enduring have been termed 'deficit symptoms' [2], while symptoms that are enduring, but have not been assessed as 'primary' or 'pseudo', have been termed 'enduring negative symptoms' [3] or 'persistently high negative symptoms' [4]. Attempts have been made to define 'caseness' by trying to identify patients suffering from a 'deficit syndrome' [2,5] or 'deficit state' [1] using combinations of diagnostic criteria, exclusion criteria (for pseudonegativity) and formal rating scales.

The negative syndrome, however defined, is not essential for diagnosis of schizophrenia, but the vast majority of patients suffer from it to some degree. The negative syndrome has been associated with developmental, structural and functional brain abnormalities, poor premorbid function and cognitive impairment. The syndrome is considered to respond inadequately to conventional neuroleptic treatment and to imply a poor prognosis and outcome. Like the disorganization syndrome, the negative syndrome is largely observed, as the patients often seem to have little insight into their deficits.

The most important negative symptoms are described below and summarized in Table 2.2. The validity of these symptomatic components within the syndrome has been implied by confirmatory factor analysis [6].

Table 2.2

\multicolumn{2}{l}{Summary of negative symptoms}	
Area	Symptoms
Affect	Decreased emotional response Vacant attitude Cold aloofness
Thought	Few ideas Simple stereotyped thoughts Reiteration and repetition
Speech	Very little speech Monosyllabic/mute
Motivation	Decreased, does nothing Loss of interest in work/leisure
Behaviour	Decreased facial expression Decreased gestures/body movements Generally slowed down
Self-care	Neglected appearance Indifferent to dirt/cold/discomfort Prompting and assistance necessary

Affect

The patient shows decreased emotional responsiveness to their surroundings and thoughts and to what people say or do to them. Affect may be flat, vacant and blunted or coarsened, or there may be a cold, aloof self-absorption. All forms of affective negative disorder result in difficulty in establishing rapport with the patient. Social disability follows, as support networks are lost because of the indifference of the patient towards relationships.

Thought/ideation

An impoverishment of thinking is discernible. The circle of ideas seems narrowed, in conversation themes are reiterated in a stereotypical and repetitive fashion without the usual elaboration. Additional cues to maintain the conversation are not forthcoming. The interviewer finds it hard to keep the conversation going and to introduce new material successfully.

Speech

The patient produces less speech and their replies are laconic and uninformative. When more severe, speech may become monosyllabic. In extreme cases, the patient is mute. As it follows from poverty of thought, poverty of speech makes maintaining the conversation difficult and unrewarding. Social interactions suffer because of this conversational deficit and the emotional unresponsiveness that goes with it; friends and eventually family tend to give up paying attention to the patient, and relationships founder as a consequence.

Motivation

The patient accomplishes little, spending long periods doing nothing, especially if no external stimulation is received. The ambitions of the patient are lost and former activities are carried out less and less, the ability to work fails, as does the motivation to pursue leisure interests. In extreme cases, the patients may need constant prompting to do even simple tasks.

Behaviour

The patient sits abnormally still. There is a blank facial expression, which does not change despite the content of conversation. There is decreased use of gesture. Body movements are reduced in number and extent, and are abnormally slow; the gait, in particular, is often lumbering and awkward. The patient takes excessive lengths of time to get anything done.

Self-care

The personal hygiene and appearance of the patient deteriorates. Patients may be malodorous with soiled, unwashed clothes worn for weeks or months. Patients may seem indifferent to dirt, cold and discomfort. In extreme cases, the patients need intensive prompting and assistance with the most basic daily activities, such as getting up, and have to be brought to the table and encouraged to eat.

References

1. Edwards J, McGorry PD, Waddell FM et al. **Enduring negative symptoms in first-episode psychosis: comparison of six methods using follow-up data.** *Schizophr Res* 1999; **40**:147–158.
2. Carpenter WT Jr, Heinrichs DW, Wagman AM. **Deficit and nondeficit forms of schizophrenia: the concept.** *Am J Psychiatry* 1988; **145**:578–583.
3. Mueser KT, Douglas MS, Bellack AS et al. **Assessment of enduring deficit and negative symptom subtypes in schizophrenia.** *Schizophr Bull* 1991; **17**:565–582.
4. McGlashan TH, Quinlan D, Galzer W et al. **Cognitive functioning and persistently high negative symptoms in chronic schizophrenia.** *Schizophr Res* 1997; **24**:115.
5. Kirkpatrick B, Buchanan RW, McKenney PD et al. **The Schedule for the Deficit Syndrome: an instrument for research in schizophrenia.** *Psychiatry Res* 1989; **30**:119–123.
6. Mortimer AM, Lund CE, McKenna PJ et al. **Rating of negative symptoms using the High Royds Evaluation of Negativity (HEN) scale.** *Br J Psychiatry Suppl* 1989; **160**:89–92.

Chapter **3**

Clinical validity of the negative syndrome

Prevalence

Assessment issues

Estimating the prevalence of the negative syndrome is complicated by a number of factors, not least the distinction between primary and pseudonegative symptoms and the need for reliability of symptom measures. Primary negative symptoms require more prolonged observation than florid positive symptoms recounted as delusions and hallucinations. Therefore, knowledge of the patient through repeated contact or through the account of an informant is important. Difficulties with the reliability of measures can be overcome by appropriate training (particularly in detecting any pseudonegative contribution), the use of suitable rating scales, and repeated measures performed in the same patients over time.

In the prodrome

It is now well recognised that the first episode of schizophrenia is almost always preceded by a prodrome of emerging and persistent changes in behaviour and functioning. Characteristic features are readily interpretable as negative symptoms, but are actually quite common in apparently 'normal' teenagers [1]. In this group, prevalences cited have been as high as 18% for 'social isolation and withdrawal', 42% for 'markedly impaired role function', 22% for 'blunted, flat or inappropriate affect', 40% for 'marked lack of initiative or energy' and 8% for 'marked impairment of personal hygiene'. These surprisingly ubiquitous features have little use in the diagnosis of schizophrenia prodromally because of their lack of specificity. Most patients established in a first episode of schizophrenia, however, do manifest them: 76% have 'social isolation and withdrawal', 63% 'markedly impaired role function', 33% 'blunted, flat or inappropriate affect' and 22% have 'marked impairment of personal hygiene'. Therefore, a group of coexisting prodromal symptoms may have some potential as an early warning sign of incipient psychosis [2]. A new scale for the detection of such a prodrome has been developed. This new scale has been validated retrospectively, but not prospectively, and is detailed in Appendix I [3].

In the first episode

The clinical picture often changes rapidly during the first episode. In addition, questions about the validity of the diagnosis and the possibility of drug abuse, as well as changes in medication, create considerable difficulties in evaluating negative symptoms at this early stage.

One solution is to identify patients who, following remission from their first episode, fulfil criteria for a 'deficit syndrome', ruling out pseudonegative symptoms from depression, Parkinsonism etc. An early study [4] found that only 12% of patients fulfilled these criteria. Another study [5] reported a similar figure, with 10% of 70 first-episode patients having a deficit syndrome on narrow criteria, but 38% fulfilling broader criteria. A third study confirmed this impression [6], with 10% of first-episode patients classified as being in a 'deficit state'. Two further studies [7,8], however, demonstrated higher prevalences of the deficit categorization (34% and 31%, respectively). Clearly, cross-study comparisons are difficult because of the lack of consensus regarding definitions and operational criteria, and variability between patient samples. A recent study [9], which used six methods of ascertaining the deficit state in 238 first-episode patients at three time points over one year, found that not only did the percentages achieving 'caseness' vary markedly according to the method used, but also that many patients crossed the threshold of caseness between assessments using the same method of ascertainment. Overall, the results were consistent with some of the earlier studies, with 9% of patients meeting a narrow definition of caseness, decreasing to 4% when exclusion criteria were applied.

In relapse
Up to 50% of people with schizophrenia undergoing acute psychotic relapse exhibit moderate-to-severe negative symptoms. These symptoms are more than likely to comprise a mixture of primary and pseudonegative symptoms; psychotic withdrawal in response to positive symptoms and the extrapyramidal side effects (EPS) of antipsychotic medication will be particularly relevant. It has been shown that during acute relapse all negative symptoms, except poverty of speech, can vary with positive symptoms, depression and side effects [10]. Furthermore, negative symptoms in acutely ill patients lack specificity to schizophrenia; they are also seen in depressive and organic states, and even in dissociative disorder. Therefore, negative symptoms in the acute state are of less diagnostic significance than the more florid positive symptoms, such as the 'first-rank symptoms' described by Schneider (eg, third-person auditory hallucinations, thought insertion and thought broadcast) [11].

Chronic patients
Residual symptoms sufficient to comprise a 'deficit state' are present in 10–12% of community-based patients with schizophrenia [12], while 50–75% of all chronic patients, wherever situated, exhibit some primary negative symptoms, with 17–25% having symptoms to a marked or severe degree [13] that are likely to be equivalent to a 'deficit state'. These residual symptoms are disease-specific (ie, they are not found in affective or other disorders after the resolution of acute episodes) [12]. One group of investigators [8,13–16] claims to have found evidence of primary negative symptoms and deficit states in patients with affective disorder, neurosis and even

personality disorder. Their methodology did not, however, allow pseudonegativity to be ruled out; negative symptom rating scales and deficit criteria alone were used without independent ratings of depression, premorbid personality, drug side effects etc. Leaving aside these criticisms, practising clinicians (as opposed to research teams) have not, as a group, identified the phenomenon of the negative syndrome in any diagnostic category except schizophrenia. Presumably, there is tacit recognition that the presentations of other groups are qualitatively different, despite some behavioural overlap.

Residual negative symptoms in people with schizophrenia are, therefore, likely to represent the primary deficit of the schizophrenic state and they are most resistant to conventional antipsychotic medication. Hence, these residual negative symptoms provide the most appropriate test of efficacy for those newer 'atypical' antipsychotic agents that purport to treat 'negative' symptoms.

Course and prognosis

From the above, it is clear that the prevalence of negative symptoms may fluctuate over time within a given schizophrenic cohort, caused by superimposed episodes of acute psychosis; however, there are primary negative symptoms that remain stable over time. For example, it has been demonstrated that most first-episode patients classified as being in a deficit state still met the criteria when readmitted [6]. This suggests that there is a degree of stability of some negative symptoms after the first episode in most patients, despite the 'moving target' nature of deficit syndrome status in its wake [9]. It has been suggested that for 40% of patients, primary negative symptoms will have emerged within the first five years of illness [14] and they may even predate the appearance of positive symptoms [17]. In first-episode patients, the severity of negative symptoms is a stronger predictor of poor quality of life two years later, than the severity of positive or disorganization symptoms [18].

Contemporary research on elderly patients who originally became ill before the neuroleptic drug era has shown that the initial duration of untreated psychosis correlates with later severity of negative symptoms [19]. Numerous studies on younger patients agree that those more severely affected are more severely ill generally and have a poorer quality of life. Premorbid associations include a longer prodrome with longer treatment delay and poorer adjustment in terms of educational achievement and social function [6,20–22]. There is no doubt that treatment delay may lead to worse clinical and social outcomes, including persistent negative symptoms [23]. It seems there is less potential for change either way in negative symptoms as the illness progresses [24,25]. There is no doubt that negative symptoms are associated with unsatisfactory personal and social function, in fact, there is a degree of circularity in that some rating scales for negative symptoms include items assessing these functions.

Does the deficit syndrome develop simply as a consequence of chronic illness or does it reflect a distinct subtype of patient? The answer may be that in some patients (comprising a subtype) an accumulation of negative symptoms is indeed a consequence of the disease process. After all, negative symptoms are not ubiquitous in patients with schizophrenia; numerous studies on samples from acute inpatients through outpatients to chronic inpatients agree that less than half of the patients suffer from negative symptoms to a marked degree [21].

What is the difference between patients predestined to manifest a deficit state and patients who will remain unaffected? Premorbid associations of deficit suggest that these patients either have a more malign disease process or are more damaged prior to the onset of the disease, or both. For example, it has been found that in male patients a history of birth complications predicts enduring negative, but not positive, symptoms [26]. It may even be the case that in some patients negative symptoms are well established prior to the point of entry into treatment. Negative symptoms can delay presentation and so become entrenched through lack of treatment. Therefore, there is an interaction between having a more severe schizophrenic illness and lengthening chronicity of untreated illness: the two are not independent in the formation of negative symptoms. Patients may have a longstanding illness, but without having reached a critical threshold of initial severity may, given appropriate treatment, avoid the development of a deficit state. These arguments are compatible with the view that the psychotic process itself may be toxic to the brain and that treatment acts to limit long-term functional impairment.

A recent study [27] investigated the increased frequency of schizophrenia in a population with learning disabilities. Structural magnetic resonance imaging (MRI) was used to compare patients with schizophrenia, patients with learning disabilities and patients with learning disabilities and comorbid schizophrenia. It was found that the scans of the comorbid group closely resembled those of the schizophrenic group, with particular similarities involving the amygdala-hippocampus. The implication is that the comorbid group are primarily patients with schizophrenia, but their disease process has been so early and so severe that it has resulted in their being diagnosed as having a learning disability. In these patients, the comorbid diagnosis of schizophrenia has arisen later, when sufficient brain development has occurred to make the manifestation of schizophrenic symptoms (presumably positive ones) possible.

Although primary symptoms probably constitute the majority of those negative symptoms persisting over long periods of time, it is worth noting the potential for change, even with a longstanding deficit. Studies of chronically institutionalized patients emerging from long stay wards in Friern and Claybury hospitals (south east England) have revealed that these people may exhibit reductions in chronic negative symptomatology when they are resettled in the community [28]. Hence, the assessment of 'true' primary negative symptoms must take into account the presence of environmental stimuli over the long term.

Relationship of the negative syndrome to affective disorder

Affective disorder, principally in the form of depression, is extremely common in schizophrenia, ranging from an insightful response to emerging disability to a genuine schizoaffective state. It is particularly common at first episode and during the first year thereafter [29]. Leaving aside the management implications, this will make negative symptoms even more difficult to assess early on in the illness. It has been found that patients with schizophrenia and a family history of affective disorder are particularly prone to developing depressive symptoms [30].

Although there is no overall correlation between depressive symptoms and negative symptoms in schizophrenia [31,32], it is possible, in factor analytic studies of major depression, to find a factor apparently identical with the negative syndrome [33]. Furthermore, it has been shown that in patients with schizophrenia, some aspects of anxiety (eg, physiological arousal) are strongly correlated with reality distortion, while some aspects of depression (eg, psychomotor slowing and loss of social interest) are related to psychomotor poverty [34]. Clearly, there is a good deal of overlap between the behavioural abnormalities in both disorders, which are simply called by different names according to diagnosis. Whether the pathophysiology is the same is open to question. While 'resting state' activity is reduced in the left prefrontal cortex in both patients with schizophrenia and depressed patients who exhibit poverty of speech (relative to those with either diagnosis that do not [35]), patients with these syndromes may differ in their ability to activate the prefrontal cortex [36]. A recent positron emission tomography (PET) study of first-episode, neuroleptic-naïve patients reported an association between depressive symptoms and lowered striatal presynaptic dopamine function. Negative symptoms were also measured, but were not significantly related to such dysfunction [37].

Antipsychotic treatment may influence depression in patients with schizophrenia. If the depression is an integral part of the schizophrenia, effective treatment of schizophrenia should cause the depression to attenuate alongside other symptoms. Although antipsychotic drugs have been traditionally used to treat depressed patients without schizophrenia, particularly where there are thought to be psychotic features, there is little evidence that these drugs are effective antidepressants in this group [38]. Furthermore, in one study of patients with chronic schizophrenia [32], the duration of antipsychotic treatment was correlated with depression despite a tendency for younger patients to be more depressed than older ones.

Relationship of negative symptoms to drug treatment

True primary symptoms are generally regarded as both longitudinally stable and unaffected by treatment with conventional antipsychotic drugs [39,40]. An attempt to find out if drug withdrawal increased primary negative symptoms, or only pseudonegative symptoms, after three-weeks' washout was unable to resolve this issue [41]; both worsened, but the ratings of primary negative symptoms only correlated with ratings of positive symptoms, not depression or side effects. It was not clear if the negative symptoms were worse because of increasing positive symptoms (ie, a pseudonegative contribution) or genuinely changing independently.

An attempted empirical validation of negative symptoms demonstrated that their factor loadings were similar whether patients were on or off medication [42]. Nevertheless, changes in motivation were predicted by alterations in anxiety and depression, while changes in affective flattening were predicted by changes in EPS. This study exemplifies the problem of differentiating true primary negative symptoms from contamination by pseudonegative symptoms owing to other causes. In keeping with this is a study of chronic hospitalized patients, which found that negative symptoms were correlated with both dose and duration of neuroleptic treatment, pointing strongly to the role of medication [32]. Since it is well known that neuroleptic drugs have little impact on negative symptoms, it is unlikely that higher doses were used for longer to treat these symptoms. A study of outpatients, however, failed to replicate this finding. Perhaps with less severe and chronic patients, raters are less inclined to attribute apparent negative symptoms to the primary category, owing to increased awareness of the overlap with side effects and depression [43].

A sensitive, reliable and valid scale for patients to rate their own subjective well-being under neuroleptic treatment has been devised; the scale measures restrictions in emotionality, 'straight thinking' and spontaneity [44]. Scores were found to improve significantly in patients switched to clozapine compared with patients remaining on conventional neuroleptic drugs. It is likely that this scale can give a good measure of pseudonegative symptoms attributable to the side effects of medication.

References

1. McGorry PD, McFarlane C, Patton GC et al. **The prevalence of prodromal features of schizophrenia in adolescence: a preliminary survey.** *Acta Psychiatr Scand* 1995; **92**:241–249.
2. Jackson HJ, McGorry PD, Dudgeon P. **Prodromal symptoms of schizophrenia in first-episode psychosis: prevalence and specificity.** *Compr Psychiatry* 1995; **36**:241–250.
3. Launer M, McKean W. **The effective management of schizophrenia within primary care.** *Prog Neurol Psychiatry* 2001; in press.
4. Husted JA, Beiser M, Iacono WG. **Negative symptoms and the early course of schizophrenia.** *Psychiatry Res* 1992; **43**:215–222.
5. Mayerhoff DI, Loebel AD, Alvir JM et al. **The deficit state in first-episode schizophrenia.** *Am J Psychiatry* 1994; **151**:1417–1422.
6. Fenton WS, McGlashan TH. **Antecedents, symptom progression, and long-term outcome of the deficit syndrome in schizophrenia.** *Am J Psychiatry* 1994; **151**:351–356.
7. Kirkpatrick B, Ram R, Bromet E. **The deficit syndrome in the Suffolk County Mental Health Project.** *Schizophr Res* 1996; **22**:119–126.

8. Gerbaldo H, Georgi K, Pieschl D. **The deficit syndrome in first-admission patients with psychotic and non-psychotic disorders.** *Eur Psychiatr* 1997; **12**:53–57.
9. Edwards J, McGorry PD, Waddell FM et al. **Enduring negative symptoms in first-episode psychosis: comparison of six methods using follow-up data.** *Schizophr Res* 1999; **40**:147–158.
10. Dollfus S, Petit M. **Negative symptoms in schizophrenia: their evolution during an acute phase.** *Schizophr Res* 1995; **17**:187–194.
11. Schneider K. *Clinical Psychopathology. 5th edition.* New York: Grune and Stratton, 1958.
12. Husted JA, Beiser M, Iacono WG. **Negative symptoms in the course of first-episode affective psychosis.** *Psychiatry Res* 1995; **56**:145–154.
13. Fenton WS, McGlashan TH. **Natural history of schizophrenia subtypes. II. Positive and negative symptoms and long-term course.** *Arch Gen Psychiatr* 1991; **48**:978–986.
14. Gerbaldo H, Helisch A, Schneider B et al. **Subtypes of negative symptoms: the primary subtype in schizophrenic and non-schizophrenic patients.** *Prog Neuropsychopharmacol Biol Psychiatry* 1994; **18**:311–320.
15. Gerbaldo H, Fickinger MP, Wetzel H et al. **Primary enduring negative symptoms in schizophrenia and major depression.** *J Psychiatr Res* 1995; **29**:297–302.
16. Gerbaldo H, Philipp M. **The deficit syndrome in schizophrenic and nonschizophrenic patients: preliminary studies.** *Psychopharmacology* 1995; **28**:55–63.
17. Hafner H, Maurer K. **Are there two types of schizophrenia? True onset and sequence of positive and negative syndromes prior to first admission.** In: *Negative Versus Positive Schizophrenia.* Edited by A Maneros, NC Andreasen and MT Tsuang. New York: Springer, 1992;134–160.
18. Ho BC, Nopoulos P, Flaum M et al. **Two-year outcome in first-episode schizophrenia: predictive value of symptoms for quality of life.** *Am J Psychiatry* 1998; **155**:1196–1201.
19. Scully PJ, Coakley G, Kinsella A et al. **Negative symptoms severity and general cognitive impairment increase with duration of initially untreated psychosis [Abstract].** *Schizophr Res* 1997; **24**:22.
20. Mueser KT, Douglas MS, Bellack AS et al. **Assessment of enduring deficit and negative symptom subtypes in schizophrenia.** *Schizophr Bull* 1991; **17**:565–582.
21. Pogue-Geile MF, Harrow M. **Negative symptoms in schizophrenia: their longitudinal characteristics and etiological hypotheses.** In: *Positive and Negative Symptoms of Psychosis: Description, Research and Future Directions.* Edited by PD Harvey and EE Walker. Hillsdale, New Jersey: Lawrence Erlbaum Associates, 1987;94–123.
22. Fennig S, Putman K, Bromet EJ et al. **Gender, premorbid characteristics and negative symptoms in schizophrenia.** *Acta Psychiatr Scand* 1995; **92**:173–177.
23. Larsen TK, Johannessen JO, Opjordsmoen S. **First-episode schizophrenia with long duration of untreated psychosis. Pathways to care.** *Br J Psychiatry Suppl* 1998; **172**:45–52.
24. Eaton WW, Thara R, Federman B et al. **Structure and course of positive and negative symptoms in schizophrenia.** *Arch Gen Psychiatry* 1995; **52**:127–134.
25. McGlashan TH, Fenton WS. **The positive-negative distinction in schizophrenia. Review of natural history validators.** *Arch Gen Psychiatry* 1992; **49**:63–72.
26. Roff JD, Knight RA. **Birth complications and subsequent negative symptoms in schizophrenia.** *Psychol Rep* 1994; **74**:635–641.
27. Johnstone EC, Best JJK, Doody GA et al. **A controlled study of the neuroanatomy of comorbid schizophrenia and learning disability.** *Schizophr Res* 1999; **36**:201–210.
28. Leff J, Thornicroft G, Coxhead N et al. **The TAPS Project. 22: a five-year follow-up of long-stay psychiatric patients discharged to the community.** *Br J Psychiatry Suppl* 1994; **165**:13–17.
29. Addington D, Addington J, Patten S. **Depression in people with first-episode schizophrenia.** *Br J Psychiatry Suppl* 1998; **172**:90–92.
30. Kendler KS, Hays P. **Schizophrenia subdivided by the family history of affective disorder. A comparison of symptomatology and course of illness.** *Arch Gen Psychiatry* 1983; **40**:951–955.
31. McKenna PJ, Lund CE, Mortimer AM. **Negative symptoms: relationship to other schizophrenic symptom classes.** *Br J Psychiatry Suppl* 1989; **155**:104–107.
32. Perenyi A, Norman T, Hopwood M et al. **Negative symptoms, depression, and parkinsonian symptoms in chronic, hospitalised schizophrenic patients.** *J Affect Disord* 1998; **48**:163–169.
33. Toomey R, Faraone SV, Simpson JC et al. **Negative, positive, and disorganised symptom dimensions in schizophrenia, major depression and bipolar disorder.** *J Nerv Ment Dis* 1998, **186**:470–476.
34. Norman RM, Malla AK, Cortese L et al. **Aspects of dysphoria and symptoms of schizophrenia.** *Psychol Med* 1998; **28**:1433–1141.

35. Dolan RJ, Bench CJ, Liddle PF et al. **Dorsolateral prefrontal cortex dysfunction in the major psychoses; symptom or disease specificity?** *J Neurol Neurosurg Psychiatry* 1993; **56**:1290–1294.
36. Berman KF, Doran AR, Pickar D et al. **Is the mechanism of prefrontal hypofunction in depression the same as in schizophrenia? Regional cerebral blood flow during cognitive activation.** *Br J Psychiatry* 1993; **162**:183–192.
37. Hietala J, Syvalahti E, Vilkman H et al. **Depressive symptoms and presynaptic dopamine function in neuroleptic-naïve schizophrenia.** *Schizophr Res* 1999; **35**:41–50.
38. Wheeler Vega JA, Mortimer AM, Tyson PJ. **Somatic treatment of psychotic depression: review and recommendations for practice.** *J Clin Psychopharmacol* 2000; **20**:504–519.
39. Crow TJ. **The two-syndrome concept: origins and current status.** *Schizophr Bull* 1985; **11**:471–486.
40. Pogue-Geile MF, Harrow M. **Negative symptoms in schizophrenia: their longitudinal course and prognostic importance.** *Schizophr Bull* 1985; **11**:427–439.
41. Miller DD, Flaum M, Arndt S et al. **Effect of antipsychotic withdrawal on negative symptoms in schizophrenia.** *Neuropsychopharmacology* 1994; **11**:11–20.
42. Kelley ME, van Kammen DP, Allen DN. **Empirical validation of primary negative symptoms: independence from effects of medication and psychosis.** *Am J Psychiatry* 1999; **156**:406–411.
43. Tugg LA, Desai D, Prendergast P et al. **Relationship between negative symptoms in chronic schizophrenia and neuroleptic dose, plasma levels and side effects.** *Schizophr Res* 1997; **25**:71–78.
44. Naber D. **A self-rating scale to measure subjective effects of neuroleptic drugs, relationships to objective psychopathology, quality of life, compliance and other clinical variables.** *Int Clin Psychopharmacol* 1995; **10**:133–138.

Chapter **4**

Neuroscience and the negative syndrome

Neuroimaging: structural

In keeping with the notion that patients with prominent negative symptoms have a more severe form of illness characterized by an irreversible pathological process [1], is the finding that a younger age of onset is associated with greater negative symptomatology. An arrest in brain development, therefore, becomes a possible candidate for this irreversible pathological process. Using computed tomographic (CT) scanning, relationships have been found between some structural parameters and impaired cognition (which is generally associated with negative symptoms) in an early onset group, but not other groups [2]. In particular, loss of asymmetry, perhaps indicating a failure to develop normal asymmetry, was present in the early onset group. A later MRI study demonstrated a left-sided increase in the sulcal space, which was specific to patients with negative symptoms [3]. It was not clear whether this was a developmental abnormality or the result of a degenerative process.

A number of postmortem studies have reported small, but significant, reductions in brain weight or volume compared with healthy control brains. It may be assumed that patients whose brains were available for postmortem study represented the most severe and chronic group who would be characterized by a high degree of negative symptoms. One study of patients whose symptoms were carefully assessed antemortem found an association between negative symptoms and brain length [4]. An MRI volumetric study of living patients [5] reported that patients with predominant negative symptoms had greater ventricle to brain ratios and sulcal cerebrospinal fluid (CSF) to brain ratios compared with both other patients and healthy control individuals. It has been difficult to demonstrate correlations between specific brain regions and negative or other symptoms [6], however, MRI studies have reported relationships with the left ventro-medial prefrontal cortex [7]. It is generally considered that deficits of cortical grey matter account for these differences.

The question is, did the brain fail to develop to its full potential size or was there loss of tissue later on as occurs in degenerative diseases such as Alzheimer's dementia? To date, there is no satisfactory answer to this question. Another possibility is that reduced brain volume is not germane to schizophrenia *per se*, but is a risk factor. One plausible suggestion [5] is that separate patterns of neuroanatomical whole-brain abnormalities, which seem to manifest themselves according to symptomatology, do reflect differential involvement of dysgenic and atrophic pathophysiological processes. An interesting recent study found that negative symptomatology 'bred true' in affected family members where the ventricular volume of the proband was expanding over time [8].

Neuroimaging: functional

The anatomy of the lateral surface of the left hemisphere is shown in Figure 4.1 and a standard brain map used for analyses of brain function is shown in Figure 4.2. Studies from neuropsychology and functional and structural brain imaging support a role for frontal lobe dysfunction in those patients with schizophrenia who are most incapacitated by negative symptoms (*see* Figures 4.3–4.5). This hypothesis is based on long-standing observations of the similarities between the effects of frontal lobe lesions in neurological patients and negative symptoms in patients with schizophrenia. The prefrontal region has been particularly implicated in the generation of actions (*see* Figure 4.6) and speech (*see* Figure 4.7) by normal healthy individuals, and hence, provides a putative substrate for dysfunction in those patients who are unable to produce spontaneous acts such as speech to a normal degree ('alogia'; *see* Figures 4.3 and 4.5 [12,14]).

Several studies have demonstrated reduced resting blood flow in the dorsolateral prefrontal cortex (DLPFC) in schizophrenia. This phenomenon seems to be associated with negative symptoms such as poverty of speech and is presumed to reflect a lack of spontaneous mental activity [10]; this finding has been replicated

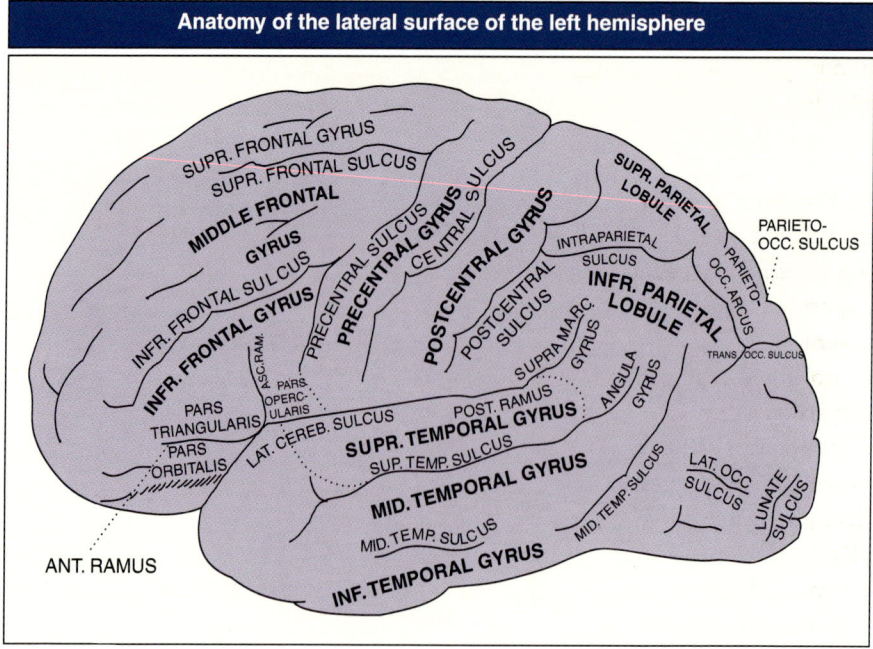

Figure 4.1. The frontal lobe is on the left of the image and the occipital lobe is to the right. The dorsolateral prefrontal cortex occupies the region of the middle and superior frontal gyri.

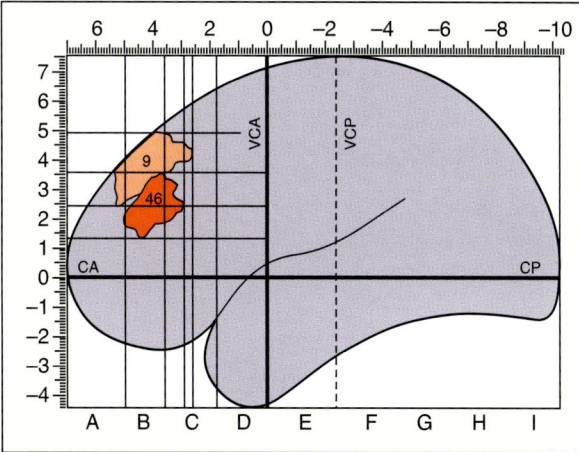

Figure 4.2. The line between CA and CP is the plane of the intercommissural line (anterior to posterior). VCA and VCP are vertical lines passing through the anterior and posterior commissures, respectively. Reproduced with permission from Rajkowska G, Goldman-Rakic PS. **Cytoarchitectonic definition of prefrontal areas in normal human cortex: II. Variability in locations of areas 9 and 46 and relationship to the Talairach Coordinate System.** *Cereb Cortex* 1995; **5**:323–337 [9].

by Ebmeier *et al.* [15] and is congruent with the findings of Suzuki *et al.* [16], relating blunted affect to the left DLPFC. A relationship has also been found between the severity of negative symptoms in unmedicated patients and prefrontal hypometabolism in the right DLPFC, which is unrelated to age, cerebral atrophy or severity of positive symptoms [17]. Elsewhere, a systematic review has discounted neuroleptic drug exposure as a simple determinant of prefrontal hypofunction [18]. Nevertheless, patients with negative symptoms may increase their DLPFC response as much as control individuals during an 'activation procedure' [19,20]. Recent studies suggest that prefrontal function may decompensate when task difficulty is increased. This phenomenon has been reported in healthy individuals [21], but is also detectable at lower task difficulty in 'deficit' patients with schizophrenia [20]. Hypofrontality has been related to performance decrement compared with control individuals on a working memory task [22]; however, this study did not rate negative symptoms specifically. It seems likely that DLPFC function is related to concurrent symptom severity in schizophrenia and that it is potentially dynamic across time [12,13].

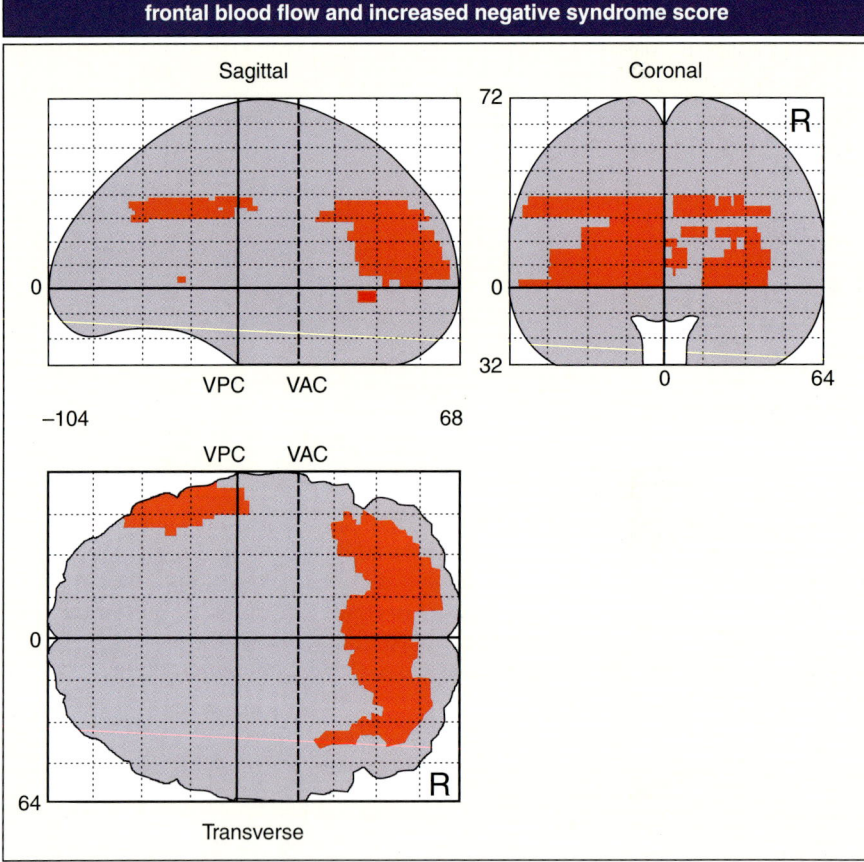

Figure 4.3. The severity of negative symptoms ('psychomotor poverty') correlated with reduced frontal blood flow. Psychomotor poverty comprises reduced speech output (alogia), affective blunting and amotivation. R, right. Reproduced with permission from Liddle PF, Friston KJ, Frith CD. **Patterns of cerebral blood flow in schizophrenia.** *Br J Psychiatry* 1992; **160**:179–186 [10].

A recent cerebral perfusion study has suggested that there may be different cerebral substrates for primary versus pseudonegative symptoms [23]: negative symptoms correlated with prefrontal hypoperfusion, while Parkinsonism correlated with the activity of the primary motor and sensory cortex. The Parkinson's disease literature, however, clearly demonstrates that this disorder may also be associated with a failure of prefrontal activation [24].

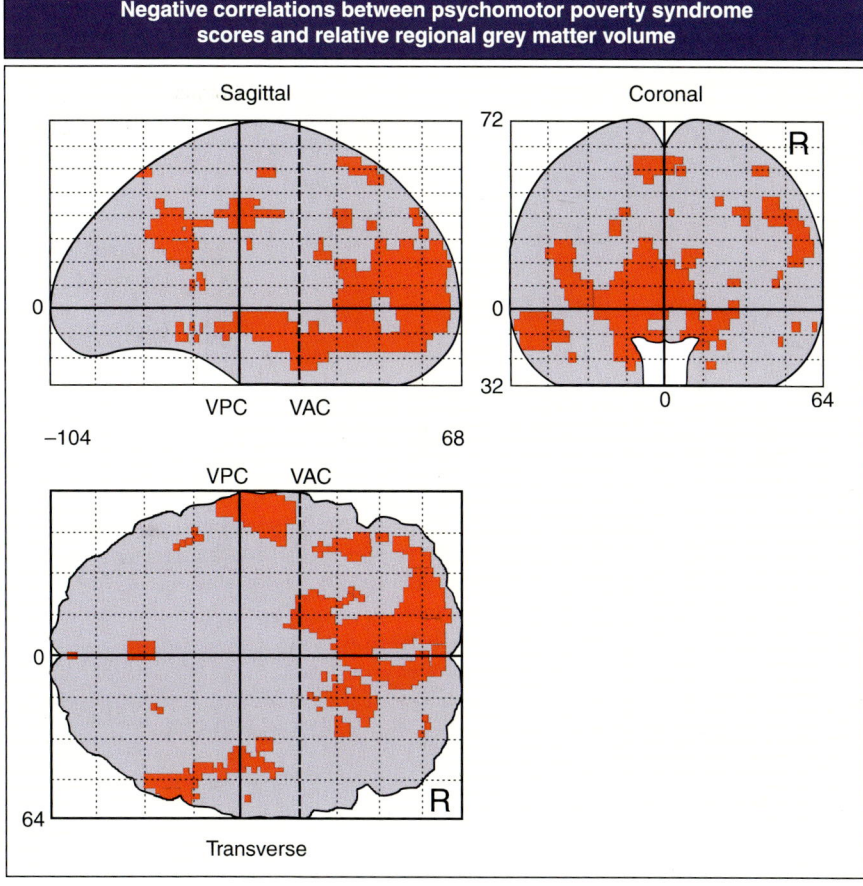

Figure 4.4. The grey matter density is reduced in the frontal lobe of patients with greater psychomotor poverty (relative to other patients with schizophrenia). R, right. Reproduced with permission from Chua SE, Wright IC, Poline JB et al. **Grey matter correlates of syndromes in schizophrenia. A semi-automated analysis of structural magnetic resonance images.** Br J Psychiatry 1997; **170**:406–410 [7].

A study in antipsychotic-naïve patients with schizophrenia has been reported [25]. In marked contrast to the above, negative symptoms significantly correlated with hypoperfusion in the left thalamic region and increased perfusion in the left frontal region. This study awaits replication.

Overall, there does seem to be a tendency for hypofrontality to be associated with the degree of negative symptomatology, at least at resting state in severely affected

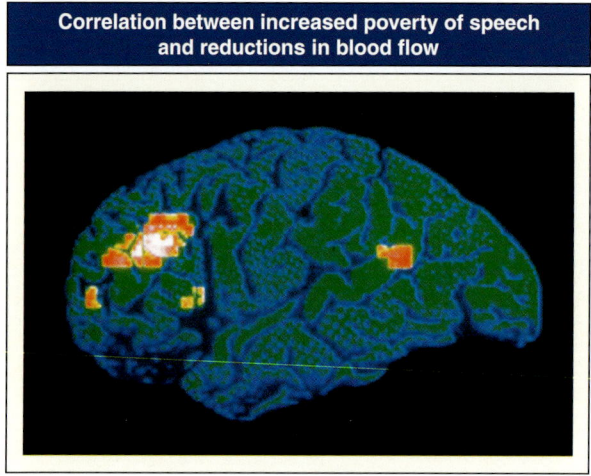

Correlation between increased poverty of speech and reductions in blood flow

Figure 4.5. The data analysis combined resting state blood flow scans from patients with schizophrenia and depression with and without poverty of speech (alogia). The authors demonstrated that independent of diagnostic category, the presence of alogia is associated with reduced blood flow in the left frontal region. The precise focus is in the left dorsolateral prefrontal cortex (Brodmann area 9). Areas highlighted indicate regions where there are significant decreases ($P < 0.01$) in regional cerebral blood flow in the poverty of speech, relative to the non-poverty, group. Data from Dolan RJ, Bench CJ, Liddle PF *et al*. **Dorsolateral prefrontal cortex dysfunction in the major psychoses; symptom or disease specificity?** *J Neurol Neurosurg Psychiatry* 1993; **56**:1290–1294 [11].

patients [10,11,15,16,26,27]. While failure to activate the prefrontal cortex may be a recurrent finding in schizophrenia, a more profound deficit may be the failure to integrate neuronal activity across this distributed brain region [13].

Neuroimaging: spectroscopy

Maier [28] has recently reviewed the spectroscopy field. Phosphorus spectroscopy may be used to assess the synthesis and breakdown of phospholipid cell membranes in the brain. Phosphomonoesters are membrane precursors, while phosphodiesters are breakdown products; the phosphomonoesters to phosphodiesters ratio gives an indication of neuronal turnover. Similarly, phosphocreatinine is a precursor in cellular energy metabolism, while inorganic phosphate is a breakdown product; the ratio of phosphocreatinine to inorganic phosphate indicates the metabolic activity of the brain.

Proton spectroscopy identifies a number of hydrogen containing molecules, some of which may be reduced where there is neuronal damage and loss. In schizophrenia,

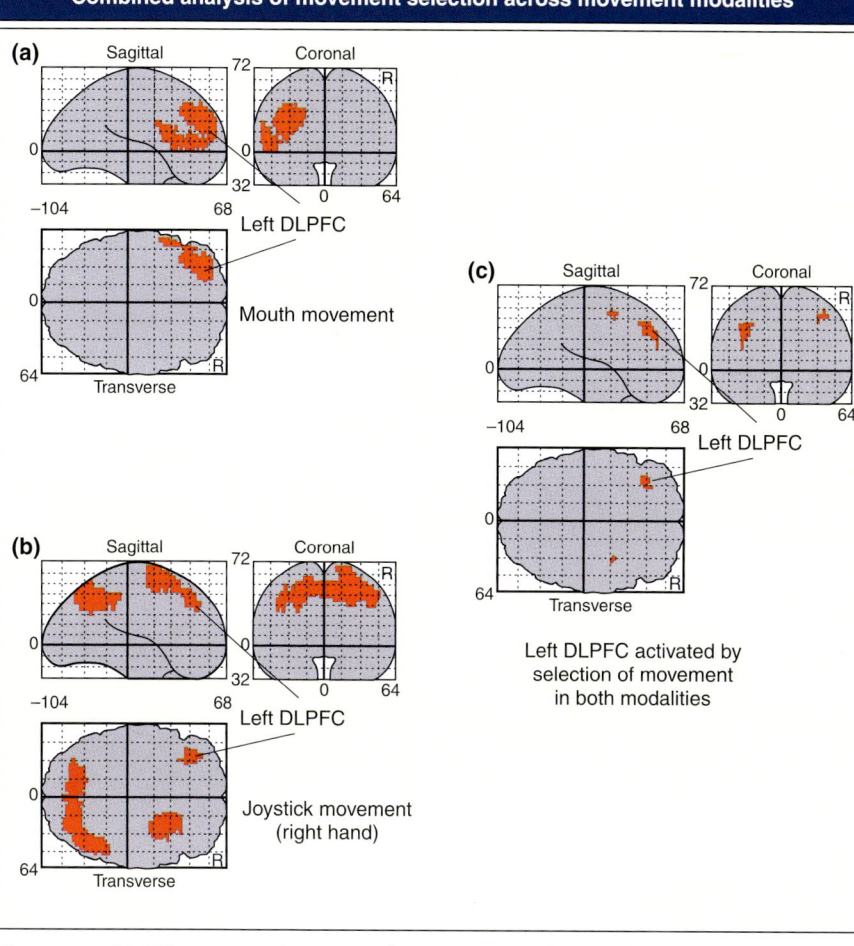

Figure 4.6. (a) When normal subjects choose to say 'lah' or 'bah' they activate the left dorsolateral prefrontal cortex (DLPFC), together with Broca's area. (b) When they choose which way to move a joystick with their right hands they also activate the left DLPFC and certain posterior brain regions concerned with spatial programming. (c) Combined analysis of these data sets reveals that left DLPFC (Brodmann area 9) is activated by choosing motor output, irrespective of its mode of output (by limb or mouth). This region is thus implicated in the self-generation of action and is the same region that was found to be underactive in those patients who exhibit reduced spontaneous speech (*see* Figure 4.5). R, right. Reproduced with permission from Spence SA, Hirsch SR, Brooks DJ *et al.* **Prefrontal cortex activity in people with schizophrenia and control subjects. Evidence from positron emission tomography for remission of 'hypofrontality' with recovery from acute schizophrenia.** *Br J Psychiatry* 1998; **172**:316–323 [12].

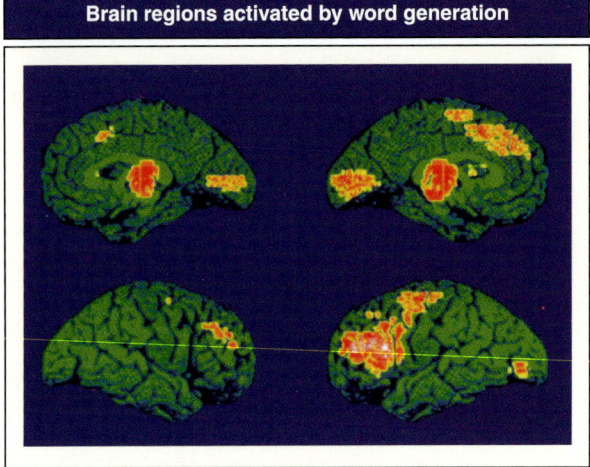

Figure 4.7. The left prefrontal cortex is maximally activated. Data from Spence SA, Liddle PF, Stefan MD et al. **Functional anatomy of verbal fluency in people with schizophrenia and those at genetic risk. Focal dysfunction and distributed disconnectivity reappraised.** *Br J Psychiatry* 2000; **176**:52–60 [13].

it has been demonstrated that drug-naïve first-episode patients have (1) decreased neuronal turnover and (2) decreased energy metabolism in the frontal lobe [29]. The former (1) is reminiscent of the picture seen in normal ageing, while the latter (2), which does not accompany the former in normal ageing, is consistent with the cerebral hypoperfusion identified in some functional imaging studies of schizophrenia. Decreased frontal neuronal turnover has been associated with the degree of negative symptoms in treated patients [30,31]. An increase in phosphocreatinine has been identified in the left frontal lobe of treated patients [32]; this suggests hypo-metabolism (thus phosphocreatinine is not being metabolised and hence, is accumulating). Evidence of neuronal damage and loss from proton spectroscopy has been reported in left medial and temporal lobes in medicated patients, but there is no association reported with negative symptoms [33].

Overall, there are some positive findings with this technique, which suggest that there is a possible degenerative process affecting relevant areas of the schizophrenic brain. There are also changes in metabolism consistent with the hypofrontality observed using other methods. Conclusive associations with negative symptoms are not yet substantiated, however, and the effects of treatment and illness chronicity are unknown, although recent preliminary findings have suggested that DLPFC neuronal integrity may be improved with antipsychotic treatment [34].

Neurochemistry

Candidate neurotransmitters and methodological problems

There are numerous neurotransmitter systems thought to be relevant to the pathophysiology of negative symptoms. The most intensively studied are the monoaminergic (noradrenaline, dopamine) and indoleaminergic (serotonin) systems. All are components of the ascending reticular-activating system (RAS), which projects from the brainstem to the forebrain and whose function is, overall, one of arousal. Arousal is clearly germane to the function of responding to stimuli and is the sum of the interplay between the neurotransmitter systems comprising the RAS. Animal work has shown that each RAS has its own tonic pattern of firing and characteristic phasic responses to various environmental stimuli such as reinforcers and noxious events. It is thought that the effect on the forebrain of increasing firing of noradrenergic and dopaminergic neurones, is to sensitize cortical regions to sensory stimuli (ie, increased signal to noise) so that arousal increases. By contrast, application of serotonin to the neocortex blunts the evoked response, a 'de-arousing' effect [35]. The other neurotransmitter thought to provide a possible substrate for the pathophysiology of negative symptoms is glutamate, which is widespread in the brain and has an excitatory function.

The meaningful study of neurotransmitter status in relation to negative symptoms is fraught with difficulty. The effects of psychotropic substances have been used to study the putative involvement of the majority of the candidate neurotransmitters. The mechanism of action of psychotropic drugs is thought to be receptor blockade of these same neurotransmitters. Therefore, any attempt to assess neurotransmitter status is subject to interference from drug treatment. Direct dynamic measures of neurotransmitter function are becoming technically possible in humans, and PET ligand studies may indicate the degree of intrinsic receptor blockade cross-sectionally. Neurotransmitter metabolites and enzymes may be quantified, but this is at the periphery and so may not accurately reflect the situation in brain tissue itself. Postmortem studies are likely to yield tissue samples subject to the effects of advanced age and significant comorbidity, alongside a lifetime's exposure to psychotropic drugs and other physical treatments. A further problem is that individual neurotransmitter systems do not act independently, but in concert; it is unlikely that a single pathology of a single population of neurones will be isolated as the core abnormality responsible for negative symptoms.

Dopamine

The dopaminergic system is thought to activate behaviour in response to cues signalling the availability of incentives or reinforcers. Behaviour activated by the dopamine system includes basic functions such as eating and drinking as well as newly learned responses. The mechanism seems to be the bringing about of a state of 'motor readiness' or response preparation, so that cues are acted upon and action occurs quickly. In addition, work with patients with Parkinson's disease whose levodopa is withdrawn, suggests that the dopaminergic system is involved in more complicated cognitive functions such as the planning and organizing of sequences of behaviour (the modulation of an 'executive network'). All the above functions have obvious relevance to negative symptomatology.

Perhaps the best indicator of dopaminergic involvement in specific symptomatology is the efficacy of conventional neuroleptic drugs, whose mechanism of action is to block the dopamine receptors and, thus, interrupt dopaminergic neurotransmission. These drugs do not improve negative symptoms [36,37], in contrast to their effects on positive symptoms (which have been hypothesized to result from an excess of dopaminergic neurotransmission). Although some studies suggest a partial improvement in negative symptoms [38–42], neuroleptic effects on pseudonegative symptoms, particularly those resulting from poorly controlled positive symptoms, cannot be ruled out. The conclusion has been drawn that pseudonegative symptoms accompanying positive symptoms in acute patients do respond to neuroleptic treatment of those positive symptoms [43].

A hypokinetic syndrome comprising anhedonia, depressed mood and cognitive impairment has been identified in patients with Parkinson's disease, retarded depression and the negative syndrome [44,45]. It is suggested that this psychopathology is identical regardless of diagnostic group, which implies a common pathophysiology involving reduced dopamine turnover. (A recent preliminary report has described an association between high dopamine-2 receptor blockade by classical antipsychotic drugs and severity of secondary depression in people with schizophrenia [46].) Further circumstantial evidence for the intrinsic involvement of dopaminergic systems, independent of drug effects, comes from the finding that Parkinsonism is common in neuroleptic-naïve first-episode patients [47–49], with up to 37% having one symptom. No association between spontaneous Parkinsonism and negative symptoms has been observed, but a small PET study of drug-naïve patients with negative symptoms has reported a high correlation between striatal dopamine receptor density and degree of negativity [50]. There is a good deal of evidence to suggest that the basal ganglia are involved in the control of motivation and cognition as well as motor function, affording them the potential to contribute to the negative syndrome [51].

Significant inverse correlations have been observed between plasma homovanillic acid (HVA), a dopamine metabolite whose levels are thought to reflect dopaminergic turnover, and negative symptom scores [52–54]. Lowered HVA excretion is seen predominantly in patients with the negative syndrome [55]. Reduced HVA levels in CSF are associated with greater ventricular to brain ratios [56–58], the latter being independently associated with negative symptoms [5]. Although neuroleptic treatment usually decreases plasma HVA by reducing dopaminergic turnover, this tends not to occur in treatment-resistant patients or those with a negative syndrome [52,53,59,60].

Dopamine transmission is facilitated by several receptors, with the dopamine-2 variety having been thought most relevant to schizophrenia. There are also inhibitory autoreceptors. Several studies suggest that the use of dopamine agonists (eg, amphetamine) improves negative symptoms such as social withdrawal, blunting of affect and motor retardation [37,61–63], but this is associated with a contemporaneous exacerbation of positive symptoms. The potential for dopamine agonism in patients with significant negative symptoms may be limited; recent research using PET suggests that negative symptoms are linked to a diminished cerebral response to dopamine [64,65]. This means that drugs that promote dopamine function through increasing levels of the neurotransmitter, decreasing its breakdown, modulating homeostatic mechanisms or stimulating target neurones in other ways, may not have as much potential for treating negative symptoms as expected. For example, the therapeutic effect of amphetamine on negative symptoms may be limited to severely affected patients, and to a modest degree only [66]. Additionally, the impaired growth hormone response to the dopamine agonist apomorphine found in patients with schizophrenia is correlated with negative symptom severity [67]. When antipsychotic treatment was withdrawn, dopamine-2 receptor availability correlated with negative symptoms [68]. Furthermore, anxiety precipitated by high doses of caffeine (a dopaminergic enhancer) in healthy control individuals was not observed in patients with schizophrenia. Although patients with schizophrenia tend to have high caffeine intakes, the idea that this could represent self-medication for negative symptoms has not been supported, since eliminating caffeine seems to have no significant effect upon these symptoms [69]. Similar arguments pertain to the excessive smoking of patients with schizophrenia [70]; stopping smoking seems to have no effect on negative symptoms [71].

Overall, there is considerable consistency in the evidence (despite its circumstantial nature and the confounding effects of treatment) for an association between diminished dopaminergic function and negative symptomatology, which fits well with the proposed roles of dopamine neurotransmission. Enhancing dopamine function directly, in order to treat these symptoms, may be problematic, however, for reasons that are currently poorly understood.

Noradrenaline
The noradrenergic system seems to have a protective function in maintaining discriminability in stressful or arousing circumstances, sustaining alertness to the most salient stimuli. This could be particularly relevant to pseudonegative symptoms resulting from poorly controlled positive symptoms. Evidence of noradrenergic abnormality related to negative symptoms is not, however, strong [72]. Reduced levels of noradrenaline and its metabolite methoxy-hydrophenylglycol (MHPG) have

been observed in the CSF of patients with negative symptoms [73], implying decreased turnover. Plasma levels, however, indicate an increase in MHPG in deficit patients, although the expected decrease in HVA was present [74]. A possible explanation is that noradrenergic neurones normally stimulate dopaminergic neurones; hence, in deficit patients there is insufficient dopaminergic response, leading to an upgrading of noradrenergic stimulation. Platelet levels of the monoamine oxidase inhibitor (MAOI), which metabolises both dopamine and noradrenaline, are, however, correlated with negative symptoms [75] and this could, in theory, lead to decreased turnover. It may be that platelet MAOI is itself upregulated, as a response to the proposed noradrenergic excess that stems from a core dopaminergic deficit in the negative syndrome.

Serotonin

A serotonin (5-hydroxytryptamine [5-HT]) hypothesis of schizophrenia predated the dopamine hypothesis; it derived from the psychotomimetic actions of the drug lysergic acid (LSD). This theory was, however, predicated on the existence of abnormal active metabolites of serotonin in patients with schizophrenia, which were conspicuous by their absence when attempts were made to find them.

Serotonin neurotransmission involves numerous receptors with different functions. In theory, an excess of serotonergic neurotransmission could produce negative symptoms; upregulation could enhance the 'de-arousing' effects of reduced signal to noise ratios produced by serotonin in the forebrain. Indicators of lower serotonin turnover have, however, been associated with negative symptoms, the opposite of what would be expected [76], although increased levels of platelet serotonin have also been found [77]. There is some evidence that the ratio between dopamine and serotonin function is more important than either transmitter alone [78]. Animal models of negative symptoms can be produced using dopamine-3-receptor agonists, which decrease serotonin turnover in the frontal cortex, but not in subcortical regions. This effect is not abolished by haloperidol (a dopamine-2-receptor antagonist), which like other conventional antipsychotic drugs is not thought to affect negative symptoms [79].

Drugs that antagonise the 5-HT-2A receptor do, however, appear to reduce negative symptoms [80,81]. Despite this finding, no alterations in these receptors have been observed in schizophrenia and as yet there is no ligand available for PET studies. Clozapine and several other atypical antipsychotic drugs do, however, induce a paradoxical internalization of the 5-HT-2A receptors in vitro and in vivo [82]. In one animal model, the glutamate antagonist, phencyclidine (*see* next page), enhances the animal version of negative symptoms, apparently through increasing serotonin turnover. Antidepressants that antagonise 5-HT-2 receptors attenuate this effect [83].

Glutamate

Glutamate neurones are ubiquitous in the brain; their general function is one of excitation. There are several different types of glutamate receptors, including the N-methyl-D-aspartate (NMDA) receptor, the alpha-amino-3-hydroxy-5-methyl-4-isoxazole-proprionic acid (AMPA) receptor, the kainate receptor and a metabotropic receptor (thought to be involved in memory). The glutamate system is an attractive candidate for central involvement in the pathophysiology of schizophrenia [84]. It is believed that the glutamate system acts as a filter to prevent the cortex being overwhelmed by sensory input (resulting in positive symptoms) and that dopaminergic pathways act to open this filter. Negative symptoms are also explicable, since it is believed that in the long-term, glutamatergic deficiency leads to excitotoxicity resulting in neuronal degeneration. This fits well with the finding that increased duration of untreated psychosis is associated with a worse outcome. Once again, direct evidence for glutamate dysfunction is variable and the relationship with negative symptoms has not been specifically addressed, but the majority of studies do support a glutamate deficiency in schizophrenia [85].

Clearly, the stage of illness and the symptom profile must be taken into consideration. At the simplest level, an increase in glutamate function would be expected early on, with the deficit showing up later in chronic deteriorated patients. One study demonstrated an association between decreases in a genetic marker for glutamate function and cognitive impairment in a postmortem sample [86]. The NMDA-receptor antagonists, phencyclidine and ketamine, can mimic both positive and negative symptoms in schizophrenia and produce animal equivalents [85], but not in immature animals or children; this is of considerable interest, given the neurodevelopmental issues in schizophrenic aetiology. Furthermore, antipsychotic drugs, but not other psychotropic medications, reduce phencyclidine-induced 'positive symptoms' in the rat model, and only atypical antipsychotic drugs reduce the rat version of 'negative symptoms'. No consistent action of antipsychotic drugs on glutamate function has been demonstrated that would explain this finding. The ability of antipsychotic drugs in development to abolish the behavioural effects of NMDA inhibition in animal models is, however, proposed as evidence that a drug should be effective against both positive and negative symptoms; in the case of olanzapine this appears to have clinical validity [87].

The NMDA receptor is a complex structure incorporating numerous modulatory sites in addition to the phencyclidine site. One such site is the sigma receptor; its natural ligands are endogenous opiates, although phencyclidine and some conventional antipsychotic drugs can also bind to it [84]. Experimental use of sigma antagonists in patients has met with mixed results. One small, open study demonstrated negative symptom improvements in some patients, although some others experienced an exacerbation in positive symptoms [88].

Neuropsychology

It is generally accepted that cognitive impairment is associated to a degree with negative symptoms, but the effects of overall severity and chronicity of illness are perhaps just as important. Whereas the primary negative syndrome may turn out to be a single entity, cognitive impairment covers a huge and diverse selection of mental functions, all of which may be assessed by a variety of tests. There are intrinsic difficulties in models of schizophrenia that try to relate specific symptoms to specific aspects of cognition [89]. Tests expected to be associated with negative symptoms must clearly reflect the concept that negative symptoms represent failure to respond to stimuli. Contamination by pseudonegativity is an obvious confounder, particularly EPS on motor or timed aspects of cognitive tasks. Even so, a degree of circularity ensues from inviting patients to display symptoms and then quantifying them with numbers; for example, lack of motivation is inevitably linked to poor test performance.

Some aspects of executive (frontal lobe) function include responding to stimuli and changing response when the stimulus changes; performance on appropriate tasks has been related to negative symptomatology perhaps more frequently than other sorts of cognitive function, such as memory [90,91]. One study reported far poorer performance on prefrontal lobe tests by patients with prominent negative symptoms, compared with patients with prominent positive symptoms [92]. Even so, there is always the danger that both poor test performance and negative symptomatology are related to prior variables of illness severity and chronicity and that the association is general rather than specific. After all, dysexecutive and negative syndromes are both common in schizophrenia. For example, one study reported that in matched samples of male and female patients the dysexecutive and negative syndromes were closely associated, but that in the women there was an increase in both with duration of illness [93]. This is compatible with the fairly well-accepted notion that schizophrenia tends to manifest as a more severe illness in men, in whom the pathology is 'locked in' earlier in its course, while in women all aspects of the disorder start off later and milder, but may worsen over time.

An attempt was made to predict the variability of negative symptoms over a one-year period in terms of initial performance on the Wisconsin Card Sorting Task [94], an accepted measure of executive function. As expected, poor performers demonstrated less variability in negative symptoms [95]. Stimulant abusers had more variability, indicating possible self-medication or simply more motivation (therefore less negative symptoms) in the first place.

One study examined an attentional task, crossover reaction time performance, in undergraduates classified as having schizoptypal personalities with various combinations of positive and negative features [96]. Negativity was related to a relative inability to benefit from regular stimulus presentation, while positive features were related to longer reaction times. Similar findings occur in patients with predominantly negative or positive symptoms. The neurophysiological basis of test performance was not discussed, but it was noted that relatives of patients with schizophrenia also perform poorly in this test. There has been interest recently in the cognitive and other characteristics of 'obligate carriers' of the genetic predisposition to schizophrenia [13,97–101]. It may be that a neurophysiological exploration of such work, focusing on relatives of deficit state patients, will eventually establish a genetic pathology of negative symptoms.

Most studies of the effects of drug treatment find that changes in cognition are unrelated to changes in symptomatology [89]. A recent study demonstrated, in clinically improved patients, independence between several cognitive functions and negative and other symptoms [102]. The association between symptoms and different aspects of performance was not easy to interpret on a simple 'failure to respond equals negative symptoms' model. For example, 'unnecessary' responses on one task were correlated with both affective flattening and hallucinations; the latter result would be predicted theoretically (as indicative of a failure to 'self-monitor'), while the former would not. If the role of the prefrontal cortex, however, incorporates both response generation and the regulation of posterior and subcortical brain regions, then it is possible to see how 'reversing' hypofrontality might lead to improvements of both negative (eg, affective flattening) and positive (eg, reality distortion) symptoms [12] and 'cognitive' impairments. The reversal of hypofrontality might, therefore, provide a means of modifying each of these impairments.

Neurophysiology

Patients with negative symptoms, but not positive symptoms, show impairment on backward masking, a measure of visual processing that is dependent on the parvocellular and magnocellular visual pathways [103]. Another visual measure, eye tracking, manifests a deficit that is correlated with negative, but not positive, symptoms [104]. Similarly, the degree of negative symptomatology is correlated with abnormalities of input processing of auditory information in the lower brainstem [105]. In college students selected for apparent subclinical negative psychopathology, but without schizophrenia at the time, there was an abnormality of evoked potentials recorded during a cognitive task involving processing of auditory information (mismatch negativity); the authors suggested that the abnormality was a result of compensatory efforts [106].

A deficit in slow-wave sleep in the form of reduced duration, particularly delta-wave counts, has been associated with increasing negative symptoms [107]. A similar association occurs with disorganization, but not reality distortion, syndrome. The deficit is thought to involve a dysfunction of frontothalamic circuits. A later study suggested that most of the difference was caused by reduced delta amplitude and that hypometabolism of the prefrontal cortex was likely to be responsible [108]; there was no relationship to neuroleptic medication. The authors pointed out that slow-wave sleep might be regulated by both the serotonin and the cholinergic systems (given their role in arousal this is not surprising); 5-HT-2A-receptor antagonists (which include some atypical neuroleptic drugs) are known to increase slow-wave sleep. Cholinergic hyperactivity has been proposed as a cause of both sleep abnormalities and negative symptoms in schizophrenia [109]. It should be noted, however, that while some atypical drugs (particularly clozapine) have anticholinergic effects, increasing anticholinergic treatment *per se* is not generally felt to be efficacious in relieving primary negative symptoms, just the 'pseudonegativity' attributable to Parkinsonism. Therefore, the neurochemical basis for the relationship of sleep abnormality to negative symptoms remains unclear, although the serotoninergic aspects and the possible relationship to hypofrontality fit well with other research.

Conclusions

A precise aetiology and pathophysiology of negative symptoms remains to be elucidated. This can be attributed to the current relatively poor understanding of normal brain function, to the practical obstacles that do not allow the direct scrutiny of malfunction in humans (hence the plethora of in vitro and animal studies) and to the difficulties in isolating primary symptoms from pseudonegativity. There is, also, the tendency to look at a single area such as neurochemistry or structure, rather than using multiple approaches in the same patient. Even so, it is hard to construe what may be the primary aetiological abnormalities as opposed to what are probably the secondary results of ensuing pathophysiology.

It seems likely that for the present the observed results of treatment approaches may be more informative than purely 'basic' neuroscientific techniques. In this respect, perhaps the most interesting findings so far relate to serotonin, glutamate and dopamine.

References

1. Crow TJ. **Molecular pathology of schizophrenia: more than one disease process?** *Br Med J* 1980; **280**:66–68.
2. Johnstone EC, Owens DG, Bydder GM *et al*. **The spectrum of structural brain changes in schizophrenia: age of onset as a predictor of cognitive and clinical impairments and their cerebral correlates.** *Psychol Med* 1989; **19**:91–103.
3. Mozley PD, Gur RE, Resnick SM *et al*. **Magnetic resonance imaging in schizophrenia: relationship with clinical measures.** *Schizophr Res* 1994; **12**:195–203.

4. Johnstone EC, Bruton CJ, Crow TJ et al. **Clinical correlates of postmortem brain changes in schizophrenia: decreased brain weight and length correlate with indices of early impairment.** *J Neurol Neurosurg Psychiatry* 1994; **57**:474–479.
5. Gur RE, Mozley PD, Shtasel DL et al. **Clinical subtypes of schizophrenia: differences in brain and CSF volume.** *Am J Psychiatry* 1995; **151**:343–350.
6. Lawrie SM, Abukmeil SS. **Brain abnormality in schizophrenia. A systematic and quantitative review of volumetric magnetic resonance imaging studies.** *Br J Psychiatry* 1998; **172**:110–120.
7. Chua SE, Wright IC, Poline JB et al. **Grey matter correlates of syndromes in schizophrenia. A semi-automated analysis of structural magnetic resonance images.** *Br J Psychiatry* 1997; **170**:406–410.
8. Filbey FM, Holcomb J, Nair TR et al. **Negative symptoms of familial schizophrenia breed true in unstable (vs. stable) cerebral-ventricle pedigrees.** *Schizophr Res* 1999; **35**:15–23.
9. Rajkowska G, Goldman-Rakic PS. **Cytoarchitectonic definition of prefrontal areas in normal human cortex: II. Variability in locations of areas 9 and 46 and relationship to the Talairach Coordinate System.** *Cereb Cortex* 1995; **5**:323–337.
10. Liddle PF, Friston KJ, Frith CD. **Patterns of cerebral blood flow in schizophrenia.** *Br J Psychiatry* 1992; **160**:179–186.
11. Dolan RJ, Bench CJ, Liddle PF et al. **Dorsolateral prefrontal cortex dysfunction in the major psychoses; symptom or disease specificity?** *J Neurol Neurosurg Psychiatry* 1993; **56**:1290–1294.
12. Spence SA, Hirsch SR, Brooks DJ et al. **Prefrontal cortex activity in people with schizophrenia and control subjects. Evidence from positron emission tomography for remission of 'hypofrontality' with recovery from acute schizophrenia.** *Br J Psychiatry* 1998; **172**:316–323.
13. Spence SA, Liddle PF, Stefan MD et al. **Functional anatomy of verbal fluency in people with schizophrenia and those at genetic risk. Focal dysfunction and distributed disconnectivity reappraised.** *Br J Psychiatry* 2000; **176**:52–60.
14. Spence SA, Frith CD. **Towards a functional anatomy of volition.** *J Consciousness Studies* 1999; **6**:11–28.
15. Ebmeier KP, Blackwood DH, Murray C et al. **Single-photon emission computed tomography with 99mTc-exametazime in unmedicated schizophrenic patients.** *Biol Psychiatry* 1993; **33**:487–495.
16. Suzuki M, Kurachi M, Kawasaki Y et al. **Left hypofrontality correlates with blunted affect in schizophrenia.** *Jpn J Psychiatry Neurol* 1992; **46**:653–657.
17. Wolkin A, Sanfilipo M, Wolf AP et al. **Negative symptoms and hypofrontality in chronic schizophrenia.** *Arch Gen Psychiatry* 1992; **49**:959–965.
18. Weinberger DR, Berman KF. **Prefrontal function in schizophrenia: confounds and controversies.** *Philos Trans R Soc Lond B Biol Sci* 1996; **351**:1495–1503.
19. Frith CD, Friston KJ, Herold S et al. **Regional brain activity in chronic schizophrenic patients during the performance of a verbal fluency task.** *Br J Psychiatry* 1995; **167**:343–349.
20. Fletcher PC, McKenna PJ, Frith CD et al. **Brain activations in schizophrenia during a graded memory task studied with functional neuroimaging.** *Arch Gen Psychiatry* 1998; **55**:1001–1008.
21. Goldberg TE, Berman KF, Fleming K et al. **Uncoupling cognitive workload and prefrontal cortical physiology: a PET rCBF study.** *Neuroimage* 1998; **7**:296–303.
22. Carter CS, Perlstein W, Ganguli R et al. **Functional hypofrontality and working memory dysfunction in schizophrenia.** *Am J Psychiatry* 1998; **155**:1285–1287.
23. Molina Rodriguez V, Montz Andree R, Perez Castejon MJ et al. **Cerebral perfusion correlates of negative symptomatology and parkinsonism in a sample of treatment-refractory schizophrenics: an exploratory 99mTc-HMPAO SPET study.** *Schizophr Res* 1997; **25**:11–20.
24. Playford ED, Jenkins IH, Passingham RE et al. **Impaired mesial frontal and putamen activation in Parkinson's disease: a positron emission tomography study.** *Ann Neurol* 1992; **32**:151–161.
25. Min SK, An SK, Jon DI et al. **Positive and negative symptoms and regional cerebral perfusion in antipsychotic-naïve schizophrenic patients: a high-resolution SPECT study.** *Psychiatry Res* 1999; **90**:159–168.
26. Bilder RM, Lipschutz-Broch L, Reiter G et al. **Intellectual deficits in first-episode schizophrenia: evidence for progressive deterioration.** *Schizophr Bull* 1992; **18**:437–448.
27. Hyde TM, Nawroz S, Goldberg TE. **Is there cognitive decline in schizophrenia? A cross-sectional study.** *Br J Psychiatry* 1994; **164**:494–500.

28. Maier M. **In vivo magnetic resonance spectroscopy. Applications in psychiatry.** *Br J Psychiatry* 1995; **167**:299–306.
29. Pettegrew JW, Keshavan MS, Panchalingram K et al. **Alterations in brain high-energy phosphate and membrane phospholipid metabolism in first-episode, drug-naïve schizophrenics. A pilot study of dorsal prefrontal cortex by in vivo phosphorus 31 nuclear magnetic resonance spectroscopy.** *Arch Gen Psychiatry* 1991; **48**:563–568.
30. Shioiri T, Kato T, Inubushi T et al. **Correlations of phosphomonoesters measured by phosphorus-31 magnetic resonance spectroscopy in the frontal lobes and negative symptoms in schizophrenia.** *Psychiatry Res* 1994; **55**:223–235.
31. Shioiri T, Someya T, Murashita J et al. **Multiple regression analysis of relationship between frontal lobe phosphorus metabolism and clinical symptoms in patients with schizophrenia.** *Psychiatry Res* 1997; **76**:113–122.
32. Kato T, Shioiri T, Murashita J et al. **Lateralized abnormality of high-energy phosphate and bilateral reduction of phosphomonoester measured by phosphorus-31 magnetic resonance spectroscopy of the frontal lobes in schizophrenia.** *Psychiatry Res* 1995; **61**:151–160.
33. Fukuzako H, Takeuchi K, Hokazono Y et al. **Proton magnetic resonance spectroscopy of the left medial temporal and frontal lobes in chronic schizophrenia: preliminary report.** *Psychiatr Res* 1995; **61**:193–200.
34. Bertolino A, Callicott JH, Elman I et al. **The effects of treatment with antipsychotics on N-acetylaspartate measures in patients with schizophrenia [Abstract].** *Schizophr Res* 2000; **41**:A219.
35. Robbins TW, Everitt BJ. **Arousal systems and attention.** In: *The Cognitive Neurosciences.* Edited by M Gazzaniga. Cambridge, MA: MIT Press, 1994;703–720.
36. Johnstone EC, Crow TJ, Frith CD et al. **Mechanism of the antipsychotic effect in the treatment of acute schizophrenia.** *Lancet* 1978; **1**:848–851.
37. Angrist B, Rotrosen J, Gershon S. **Differential effects of amphetamine and neuroleptics on negative vs. positive symptoms of schizophrenia.** *Psychopharmacology (Berl)* 1980; **72**:17–19.
38. Goldberg SC, Schooler NR, Mattsson N. **Paranoid and withdrawal symptoms in schizophrenia: differential symptom reduction over time.** *J Nerv Ment Dis* 1967; **145**:158–162.
39. Goldberg SC. **Negative and deficit symptoms in schizophrenia do respond to neuroleptics.** *Schizophr Bull* 1985; **11**:453–456.
40. van Kammen DP, Hommer DW, Mallas KL. **Effect of pimozide on positive and negative symptoms in schizophrenic patients: are negative symptoms state dependent?** *Neuropsychobiology* 1987; **18**:113–117.
41. Breier A, Wolkowitz OM, Doran AR et al. **Neuroleptic responsivity of negative and positive symptoms in schizophrenia.** *Am J Psychiatry* 1987; **144**:1549–1555.
42. Tandon R, Goldman RS, Goodson J et al. **Mutability and relationship between positive and negative symptoms during neuroleptic treatment in schizophrenia.** *Biol Psychiatry* 1990; **27**:1323–1326.
43. Moller HJ. **Neuroleptic treatment of negative symptoms in schizophrenic patients. Efficacy problems and methodological difficulties.** *Eur Neuropsychopharmacol* 1993; **3**:1–11.
44. Hoffman WF, Labs SM, Casey DE. **Neuroleptic-induced parkinsonism in older schizophrenics.** *Biol Psychiatry* 1987; **22**:427–439.
45. Prosser ES, Csernansky JG, Kaplan J et al. **Depression, parkinsonian symptoms, and negative symptoms in schizophrenics treated with neuroleptics.** *J Nerv Ment Dis* 1987; **175**:100–105.
46. Bressan RA, Bigliani VB, Mulligan RS et al. **Striatal D_2 blockade and depression in schizophrenia: preliminary SPET findings [Abstract].** *Schizophr Res* 2000; **41**:A238.
47. Caligiuri M, Lohr JB, Jeste DV. **Parkinsonism in neuroleptic naïve schizophrenic patients.** *Am J Psychiatry* 1993; **150**:1343–1348.
48. McCreadie RG, Thara R, Kamath S et al. **Abnormal movements in never-medicated Indian patients with schizophrenia.** *Br J Psychiatry* 1996; **168**:221–226.
49. Kopala LC, Good KP, Honer WG. **Extrapyramidal signs and clinical symptoms in first-episode schizophrenia: response to low-dose risperidone.** *J Clin Psychopharmacol* 1997; **17**:308–313.
50. Martinot JL, Paillère-Martinot ML, Loc'h C et al. **Central D_2 receptors and negative symptoms of schizophrenia.** *Br J Psychiatry* 1994; **164**:27–34.
51. Graybiel AM. **The basal ganglia and cognitive pattern generators.** *Schizophr Bull* 1997; **23**:459–469.

52. Davila DG, Menero E, Zumarraga AI et al. **Plasma homovanillic acid as a predictor of response to neuroleptics [Abstract].** Arch Gen Psychiatry 1988; **45**:567.
53. Angrist R, Powchick P, Warne PA et al. **Measurement of plasma homovanillic acid concentrations in schizophrenic patients.** Prog Neuropsychopharmacol Biol Psychiatry 1990; **14**:271–287.
54. Steinberg JL, Garver DL, Moeller FG et al. **Serum homovanillic acid levels in schizophrenic patients and normal control subjects.** Psychiatry Res 1993; **48**:93–106.
55. Mathieu P, Lemoine P, Szestak M et al. **Homovanillic acid (HVA) urinary excretion and day/night rhythm of chronic schizophrenic patients. Preliminary observations.** Encephale 1985; **11**:199–202.
56. Nyback H, Berggren BM, Hindmarsh T et al. **Cerebroventricular size and cerebrospinal fluid monoamine metabolites in schizophrenic patients and healthy volunteers.** Psychiatry Res 1983; **9**:301–308.
57. Lindstrom LH. **Low HVA and normal 5HIAA CSF levels in drug-free schizophrenic patients compared to healthy volunteers: correlations to symptomatology and family history.** Psychiatry Res 1985; **14**:265–273.
58. Losonczy MF, Song IS, Mohs RC et al. **Correlates of lateral ventricular size in chronic schizophrenia, II: biological measures.** Am J Psychiatry 1986; **143**:1113–1118.
59. Pickar D, Labarca R, Doran AR et al. **Longitudinal measurement of plasma homovanillic acid levels in schizophrenic patients. Correlation with psychosis and response to neuroleptic treatment.** Arch Gen Psychiatry 1986; **43**:669–676.
60. Duncan E, Wolkin A, Angrist B et al. **Plasma homovanillic acid in neuroleptic responsive and non-responsive schizophrenics.** Biol Psychiatry 1993; **34**:535–528.
61. Angrist B, Peselow E, Rubinstein M et al. **Partial improvement in negative schizophrenic symptoms after amphetamine.** Psychopharmacology (Berl) 1982; **78**:128–130.
62. Lieberman JA, Kane JM, Gadaletta D et al. **Methylphenidate challenge tests and course of schizophrenia.** Psychopharmacol Bull 1985; **21**:123–129.
63. van Kammen DP, Boronow JJ. **Dextro-amphetamine diminishes negative symptoms in schizophrenia.** Int Clin Psychopharmacol 1988; **3**:111–121.
64. Abi-Dargham A, Gli R, Krystal J et al. **Increased striatal dopamine transmission in schizophrenia: confirmation in a second cohort.** Am J Psychiatry 1998; **155**:761–767.
65. Wolkin A, Sanfilipo M, Duncan E et al. **Blunted change in cerebral glucose utilization after haloperidol treatment in schizophrenic patients with prominent negative symptoms.** Am J Psychiatry 1996; **153**:346–354.
66. Sanfilipo M, Wolkin A, Angrist B et al. **Amphetamine and negative symptoms of schizophrenia.** Psychopharmacology (Berl) 1996; **123**:211–214.
67. Ferrier IN, Crow TJ, Roberts GW et al. **Clinical effects of apomorphine in schizophrenia.** In: Psychopharmacology of the Limbic System. Edited by M Trimble and E Zarafian. Oxford: Oxford University Press, 1984.
68. Knable MB, Egan MF, Heinz A et al. **Altered dopaminergic function and negative symptoms in drug-free patients with schizophrenia. [^{123}I]-iodobenzamide SPECT study.** Br J Psychiatry 1997; **171**:574–577.
69. Hughes JR, McHugh P, Holtzman S. **Caffeine and schizophrenia.** Psychiatr Serv 1998; **49**:1415–1417.
70. Forchuk C, Norman R, Malla A et al. **Smoking and schizophrenia.** J Psychiatr Ment Health Nurs 1997; **4**:355–359.
71. Addington J, el-Guebaly N, Campbell W et al. **Smoking cessation treatment for patients with schizophrenia.** Am J Psychiatry 1998; **155**:974–976.
72. Rao ML, Moller HJ. **Biochemical findings of negative symptoms in schizophrenia and their putative relevance to pharmacologic treatment. A review.** Neuropsychobiology 1994; **30**:160–172.
73. van Kammen DP, Mouton A, Kelley ME et al. **Explorations of dopamine and noradrenaline activity and negative symptom on schizophrenia: concepts and controversies.** In: Negative Versus Positive Schizophrenia. Edited by A Maneros, NC Andreason and MT Tsuang. Berlin: Springer, 1991;317–340.
74. Thibaut F, Ribeyre JM, Dourmap N et al. **Plasma 3-methoxy-4-hydroxyphenylglycol and homovanillic acid measurements in deficit and nondeficit forms of schizophrenia.** Biol Psychiatry 1998; **43**:24–30.
75. Lewine RJ, Meltzer HY. **Negative symptoms and platelet monoamine oxidase activity in male schizophrenic patients.** Psychiatry Res 1984; **12**:99–109.
76. Pivac N, Muck-Seler D, Jakovljevic M. **Platelet 5-HT levels and hypothalamic-pituitary-adrenal axis activity in schizophrenic patients with positive and negative symptoms.** Neuropsychobiology 1997; **36**:19–21.

77. Bleich A, Brown SL, Kahn R et al. **The role of serotonin in schizophrenia.** *Schizophr Bull* 1988; **14**:297–315.
78. Meltzer HY. **The role of serotonin in antipsychotic drug action.** *Neuropsychopharmacology* 1999; **21**:106S–115S.
79. Lynch MR. **Selective effects on prefrontal cortex serotonin by dopamine D3 receptor agonism: interaction with low-dose haloperidol.** *Prog Neuropsychopharmacol Biol Psychiatry* 1997; **21**:1141–1153.
80. Schmidt CJ, Sorensen SM, Kehne JH et al. **The role of 5-HT2A receptors in antipsychotic activity.** *Life Sci* 1995; **56**:2209–2222.
81. Leysen JE, Gommeren W, Schotte A. **Serotonin receptor subtypes: possible roles and implications in antipsychotic drug action.** In: *Serotonin in Antipsychotic Treatment.* Edited by JM Kane, H Moller and F Awouters. New York: Marcel Dekker, 1996;51–75.
82. Willins DL, Berry SA, Alsayegh L et al. **Clozapine and other 5-hydroxytryptamine-2A receptor antagonists alter the subcellular distribution of 5-hydroxytryptamine-2A receptors in vitro and in vivo.** *Neuroscience* 1999; **91**:599–606.
83. Noda Y, Mamiya T, Furukawa H et al. **Effects of antidepressants on phencyclidine-induced enhancement of immobility in a forced swimming test in mice.** *Eur J Pharmacol* 1997; **324**:135–140.
84. Carlsson A, Hansson LO, Waters N et al. **A glutamatergic deficiency model of schizophrenia.** *Br J Psychiatry Suppl* 1999; **174**:2–6.
85. Sams-Dodd F. **Phencyclidine in the social interaction test: an animal model of schizophrenia with face and predictive validity.** *Rev Neurosci* 1999; **10**:59–90.
86. Humphries C, Mortimer A, Hirsch S et al. **NMDA receptor mRNA correlation with antemortem cognitive impairment in schizophrenia.** *Neuroreport* 1996; **7**:2051–2055.
87. Moore NA. **Olanzapine: preclinical pharmacology and recent findings.** *Br J Psychiatry Suppl* 1999; **37**:41–44.
88. Modell S, Naber D, Holzbach R. **Efficacy and safety of an opiate sigma-receptor antagonist (SL 82.0715) in schizophrenic patients with negative symptoms: an open dose-range study.** *Pharmacopsychiatry* 1996; **29**:63–66.
89. Mortimer AM. **The neuropsychology of schizophrenia.** In: *The Psychopharmacology of Schizophrenia.* Edited by JFW Deakin and MA Reveley. London: Arnold, 2000;153–177.
90. Frith CD, Leary J, Cahill C et al. **Performance on psychological tests. Demographic and clinical correlates of the results of these tests.** *Br J Psychiatry Suppl* 1991; **159**:26–29.
91. Voruganti LN, Heslegrave RJ, Awad AG. **Neurocognitive correlates of positive and negative syndromes in schizophrenia.** *Can J Psychiatry* 1997; **42**:1066–1071.
92. Mattson DT, Berk M, Lucas MD. **A neuropsychological study of prefrontal lobe function in the positive and negative subtypes of schizophrenia.** *J Genet Psychol* 1997; **158**:487–494.
93. Scully PJ, Coakley G, Kinsella A et al. **Executive (frontal) dysfunction and negative symptoms in schizophrenia: apparent gender differences in 'static' v. 'progressive' profiles.** *Br J Psychiatry* 1997; **171**:154–158.
94. Milner B. **Effects of different brain lesions on card sorting.** *Arch Neurol* 1963; **9**:90–100.
95. Lysaker PH, Bell MD, Bioty SM et al. **Cognitive impairment and substance abuse history as predictors of the temporal stability of negative symptoms in schizophrenia.** *J Nerv Ment Dis* 1997; **185**:21–26.
96. Sarkin AJ, Dionisio DP, Hillix WA et al. **Positive and negative schizotypal symptoms relate to different aspects of crossover reaction time task performance.** *Psychiatry Res* 1998; **81**:241–249.
97. Honer WG, Bassett AS, Squires-Wheeler E et al. **The temporal lobes, reversed asymmetry and the genetics of schizophrenia.** *Neuroreport* 1995; **7**:221–224.
98. Frangou S, Sharma T, Alarcon G et al. **The Maudsley Family Study, II: endogenous event-related potentials in familial schizophrenia.** *Schizophr Res* 1997; **23**:45–53.
99. Deakin FW, Simpson MD, Slater P et al. **Familial and developmental abnormalities of frontal lobe function and neurochemistry in schizophrenia.** *J Psychopharmacol* 1997; **11**:133–142.
100. Sharma T, du Boulay G, Lewis S et al. **The Maudsley Family Study, I: structural brain changes on magnetic resonance imaging in familial schizophrenia.** *Prog Neuropsychopharmacol Biol Psychiatry* 1997; **21**:1297–1315.
101. Sharma T, Lancaster E, Lee D et al. **Brain changes in schizophrenia. Volumetric MRI study of families multiply affected with schizophrenia – the Maudsley Family Study 5.** *Br J Psychiatry* 1998; **173**:132–138.

102. Suslow T, Junghanns K, Weitzsch C et al. **Relations between neuropsychological vulnerability markers and negative symptoms in schizophrenia.** *Psychopathology* 1998; **31**:178–187.

103. Slaghuis WL, Curran CE. **Spatial frequency masking in positive- and negative-symptom schizophrenia.** *J Abnorm Psychol* 1999; **108**:42–50.

104. Roitman SE, Keefe RS, Harvey PD et al. **Attentional and eye tracking deficits correlate with negative symptoms in schizophrenia.** *Schizophr Res* 1997; **26**:139–146.

105. Igata M, Ohta M, Hayashida Y et al. **Missing peaks in auditory brainstem responses and negative symptoms in schizophrenia.** *Jpn J Psychiatry Neurol* 1994; **48**:571–578.

106. Fernandes LO, Keller J, Giese-Davis JE et al. **Converging evidence for a cognitive anomaly in early psychopathology.** *Psychophysiology* 1999; **36**:511–521.

107. Keshavan MS, Miewald J, Haas G et al. **Slow-wave sleep and symptomatology in schizophrenia and related psychotic disorders.** *J Psychiatr Res* 1995; **29**:303–314.

108. Kajimura N, Kato M, Okuma T et al. **Relationship between delta activity during all-night sleep and negative symptoms in schizophrenia: a preliminary study.** *Biol Psychiatry* 1996; **39**:451–454.

109. Tandon R. **Cholinergic aspects of schizophrenia.** *Br J Psychiatry Suppl* 1999; **174**:7–11.

Chapter **5**

The burden of negative symptoms

Impact on the individual and their family

There is no doubt that negative symptoms are associated with a high degree of functional impairment [1]. They also constitute a risk factor for disfiguring tardive dyskinesia, particularly if accompanied by old age and Parkinsonism [2].

Many patients with pronounced negative symptoms seem unaware of their deficits and they may fail to appreciate the severity of their social implications. Hence, they may be at particular risk of self-neglect, physical illness, exploitation by others and eventual homelessness should they 'fall through the net' of community care. It has been reported that lack of motivation is the most important schizophrenic symptom in predicting quality of life at follow-up after relapse [3].

Lack of insight may be a cause of suffering to the families and carers of patients, through changed behaviour, lack of concern, possible coarsening of conduct and language or a risk of fire (through failure to extinguish lighted cigarettes). To those who do not know them, such patients may appear bizarre or threatening; they may be stigmatized because of their dishevelled appearance. One study suggested that the main concerns identified by families were not positive symptoms, but negative symptoms (particularly social withdrawal, lack of communication skills, poor social skills, decreased motivation, excessive sleeping and poor hygiene and personal habits) [4]. It is possible that negative symptoms create more problems in families than positive symptoms because the former are more likely to be overlooked in treatment, and less likely to be improved by medication.

The majority of patients with schizophrenia are smokers, up to 88% in some studies [5]. Nicotine has complex neurotransmitter effects including dopaminergic enhancement, which might, theoretically, ameliorate negative symptoms and reduce Parkinsonian side effects, and could explain the reason for heavy smoking in these patients. The burden of expense, damage to physical health and inconvenience and unpleasantness for others, particularly families, however, must be set against this.

Patients with severe negative symptoms usually have problems engaging with therapeutic programmes and may need to be prompted in the everyday tasks of self-care and hygiene. Because of their withdrawal from social contact they may be difficult to interest initially. Some tolerance on the part of community-based staff may be required for long periods before patients begin to engage, albeit in a limited way. Nevertheless, the impact of some modern treatments upon some of these patients can be momentous, leading to emergence from chronic psychosis and withdrawal. In the authors' experience this can cause problems of its own, in terms of understandable depressive reactions resulting from insight about disability, loss of relationships and career prospects.

Economic burden

The economic burden of schizophrenia is spread among patients, their families and society in general. It includes the cost of caring for patients in hospitals and hostels, the cost of prescribing antipsychotic medication and the loss of earning potential, both in patients and those members of their families who may stay at home to care for them. The cost of community care is likely to escalate as hospital beds are closed; alternative resources should include staff teams and facilities that are able to adapt flexibly to providing care in the community. 'Outreach' nurses, 'crisis intervention' teams, 'drop-in' centres and the whole range of minimally-to-intensively supported hostel accommodation, provided both by statutory and voluntary sectors, will be necessary. Other costs accrue, which are more difficult to assess; the cost of patients involved with the criminal justice system, the cost of allied medical conditions (respiratory and cardiovascular disease) and the 'opportunity cost' when resources are diverted towards the treatment of schizophrenia at the expense of other psychiatric or medical disorders.

In the UK in the early 1990s, the total 'direct' cost of treating schizophrenia was £397 million per annum (1.6% of the total healthcare budget). Drugs accounted for 5% of this cost, while hospital and community-based residential care accounted for nearly 75%. Davies and Drummond [6] estimated the indirect costs of lost production to be £1.7 billion, which was a 'conservative estimate'. More importantly, the clinical heterogeneity of schizophrenia meant that the cost of the disease was not distributed evenly among patients with the diagnosis. Of the direct costs, 97% were incurred by less than 50% of the patients. Hence, 'treatments that reduce the dependence and disability of those most severely affected by schizophrenia are likely to have a large effect on the total cost of the disease to society and may, therefore, be cost-effective, even though they appear expensive initially' [6].

Because most of the cost of schizophrenia to society attaches to those with the most severe symptomatology (likely to include those with the most negative symptoms), that cost is most sensitive to changes in the proportion of patients who fall into the most severe outcome categories (ie, the proportion who are most impaired by their symptoms). A treatment that improves outcome in even a small percentage of this severely affected group would, therefore, have a disproportionate effect upon the cost of schizophrenia to society (and hopefully a beneficial effect upon the lives of those individuals concerned). For example, the use of clozapine in treatment-resistant schizophrenia would be cost effective if it permitted discharge of at least 16% of such patients from institutions, despite the fact that a year's prescription of clozapine costs approximately seven times that of a conventional neuroleptic drug [6].

References

1. Palcios-Araus L, Herran A, Sandoya M et al. **Analysis of positive and negative symptoms in schizophrenia. A study from a population of long-term outpatients.** *Acta Psychiatr Scand* 1995; **92**:178–182.
2. Yuen O, Caligiuri MP, Williams R et al. **Tardive dyskinesia and positive and negative symptoms of schizophrenia. A study using instrumental measures.** *Br J Psychiatry* 1996; **168**:702–708.
3. Bow-Thomas CC, Velligan DI, Miller AL et al. **Predicting quality of life from symptomatology in schizophrenia at exacerbation and stabilization.** *Psychiatry Res* 1999; **86**:131–142.
4. North CS, Pollio DE, Sachar B et al. **The family as caregiver: a group psychoeducation model for schizophrenia.** *Am J Orthopsychiatry* 1998; **68**:39–46.
5. Forchuk C, Norman R, Malla A et al. **Smoking and schizophrenia.** *J Psychiatr Ment Health Nurs* 1997; **4**:355–359.
6. Davies LM, Drummond MF. **Economics and schizophrenia: the real cost.** *Br J Psychiatry Suppl* 1994; **165**:18–21.

Chapter 6

Assessment of negative symptoms

Primary and pseudonegative symptoms

It seems likely that the core deficits in the negative syndrome are poverty of affect and poverty of ideation. Given the lack of capacity to respond to one's surroundings and the people in them and the lack of internal stimulation from one's own thoughts, it is easy to see how drive, motor behaviour, and social and personal function can become compromised. These aspects of the negative syndrome are, thus, truly secondary to the primary core deficits in affect and ideation.

One result of negative symptom research has been to highlight the differential diagnosis of apparent negative symptoms (ie, the existence of pseudonegative symptoms). Pseudonegative symptoms result from unresolved positive symptoms, Parkinsonian side effects, oversedation, depression, premorbid personality traits and the effects of an institutional environment. The presentation of pseudonegative symptoms differs substantially from those of primary symptoms, in that the former are likely to be transitory, variable, or both, depending on cause and severity; they will also be accompanied by specific manifestations of the underlying cause. True negative symptoms are attributable to the pathophysiology of schizophrenia itself, are relatively stable and closely associated with each other.

A large study of the reliability of distinguishing primary from pseudonegative symptoms found poor agreement between untrained raters, who apparently under-rated pseudonegative symptoms, but yet professed high confidence in the adequacy of the information underlying their evaluations [1]. Special training in making these distinctions, the development of sophisticated rating instruments, or both, was thought necessary for valid assessments to be made. This issue is crucial for patients; negative symptoms of whatever type are burdensome, but pseudonegative symptoms should be at least partially treatable.

Presence and severity: clinical assessment versus rating scale assessment

Negative symptoms are assessed during the course of the ordinary clinical interview by using careful observation to detect their presence. An informant is often useful, especially when the patient is unforthcoming about such issues as their daily activities.

Several rating scales are available for the assessment of severity, some of which are reproduced in Appendices II–VI. The scales range from a few items drawn from general psychopathology instruments (Brief Psychiatric Rating Scale [BPRS] [2], Krawiecka scale [3,4]) to longer, complex inventories designed to cover all possible kinds of negative symptoms (High Royds Evaluation of Negativity [HEN] [5], SANS [6], Positive and Negative Syndromes of Schizophrenia [PANSS] negative subscale [7]). The longer instruments are used in research, particularly into the effects of drug treatments on negative symptoms. They are of limited clinical use when compared with the application of skilled observation and interpretation of the overall presentation and behaviour of the patient; however, training in the use of these rating scales is valuable in learning these clinical skills.

Advantages and disadvantages of the longer instruments include the following:

- The PANSS negative scale has items that are predominantly on the core symptoms of poverty of affect and ideation, which avoids rating secondary handicaps such as poor self-care. The scale does not rate motor behaviour, which most psychiatrists would consider relevant to severity. Poverty of affect is difficult to rate reliably and objectively. The scale has only seven items, but each has seven anchor points and it is not possible to score zero even if healthy.
- The SANS scale is probably the best-known scale and has been used in numerous studies. It is, however, rather long, relies on an informant and tries to assess the patient's own insight, which is often lacking. The original version includes an item on inappropriate affect, which is no longer considered to be a negative symptom (it is a feature of the disorganization syndrome).
- The HEN scale uses core symptoms that are not weighted, but it is comprehensive in addressing all aspects of primary symptoms and there is no need for an informant for most of the items. There are 24 items with four simple anchor points, which makes it fast and easy to use.

Appraisal of clinical trial results

It should be noted that no scale is able to distinguish true negative symptoms from pseudonegative symptoms attributable to independent causes; accurate differential diagnosis of the patient's presentation is crucial. A consensus paper on the assessment of negative symptoms for clinical trials recommended that patients should have had negative symptoms for at least six months; depressive, extrapyramidal and positive symptoms should be at low levels at baseline and should be measured during the study. The trials should be placebo-controlled, randomized and double-blind, lasting at least eight weeks and a global clinical impression scale should also be used [8]. Placebo control, however, causes some problems of interpretation in that it does not translate readily to real life, in which the clinician needs to choose between real treatments (when researching atypical drugs, ideally a conventional neuroleptic comparator would be more useful).

Differential diagnoses and their management

Uncontrolled positive symptoms

Patients who are withdrawn owing to preoccupation with positive symptoms may appear to have negative symptoms. Useful clues include inappropriate affect, fragments of thought disorder, abnormal involuntary movements, hallucinatory behaviour and an affect that is guarded and suspicious rather than flat. The vacant, indifferent quality to presentation is missing and the patient may appear puzzled or in a dream-like state. Social withdrawal is usually active rather than passive and there may be verbal or physical outbursts. The patient should respond to more effective antipsychotic treatment continued for adequate lengths of time.

Parkinsonism

Nearly all conventional neuroleptic drugs cause EPS in most patients [9]. Parkinsonian side effects are a common form of EPS. Such side effects, especially a mask-like face and bradykinesia, are easily mistaken for real negative symptoms. The Parkinsonism scores of patients taking haloperidol, but not of patients taking the relatively EPS-free atypical drug olanzapine, predicted a high proportion of the variance in negative symptoms [10]. Other Parkinsonian phenomena should be assessed; including tremor, rigidity, sialorrhoea, festinant gait with simian arm posture and micrographia. The patient will respond to anticholinergic medication such as benzhexol, but this can antagonise the antipsychotic effects of neuroleptic drugs [11,12]. Anticholinergic drugs can be addictive and long-term use is not recommended [13]. A reduction of the dose of antipsychotic drugs should always be attempted or a switch to a lower potency drug that does not have a high affinity for dopamine receptors. The new atypical antipsychotic drugs, which have a mild side effect profile (eg, risperidone, olanzapine and quetiapine), are an increasingly popular choice.

Oversedation and fatigue

Oversedated patients often have little drive, but complain about it or appear drowsy or sleep for long periods. It is important to rule out medical causes of fatigue, such as an endocrine disorder, anaemia etc. Antipsychotic drugs known to produce sedation as a frequent side effect include low-potency neuroleptic drugs (eg, chlorpromazine) and some atypical drugs (eg, olanzapine). If alternative drugs cannot be used, they should be given at night in the smallest possible dose. Many patients are prescribed other drugs such as sedating antidepressants and benzodiazepines, and it may be possible to reduce or stop these drugs.

Patients, especially those on conventional treatment, frequently complain of feeling 'drugged up', unable to concentrate or 'like a zombie' [14]. Such patients present as lacking motivation, being lethargic and emotionally unresponsive. It is likely that there is a mixture of what is probably an experience of oversedation, with elements of Parkinsonism and also depression or dysphoria [15]. This syndrome is known as the 'neuroleptic-induced deficit syndrome' [16]. The usual clinical 'rules of thumb' apply when it is felt that the apparent negative symptoms of the patient are a manifestation of this neuroleptic-induced deficit syndrome; the lowest effective dose of the best-tolerated effective antipsychotic should be used, any polypharmacy should be rationalized, and the doses should be once daily at night, etc.

Depression

Patients with depression who are retarded in motor behaviour and who say and do little may be misdiagnosed as having schizophrenia on the grounds of an apparent negative syndrome. Patients with depression can be encouraged, however, to describe their low mood and will usually convey distress, whereas the patient with a truly flat affect will maintain indifference. Other useful clues are diurnal variation of mood, early wakening, depressive ideation, recent onset of anhedonia, suicidal ideation, etc. Although there is no correlation between depression and negative symptoms in schizophrenia, genuine depressive symptoms are very common in patients with schizophrenia. These range from an insightful response to emerging disability, to an authentic schizoaffective state. There is little conclusive literature on effective treatment for depression in schizophrenia, but it would seem sensible for management to be informed by what is known about patients with depression without schizophrenia, plus an appraisal of the relevance of the psychotic illness in that individual. It is most important to evaluate the cause of the low mood: is it understandable misery or is the mood disproportionate to the life situation? Can the depression be construed as part of the illness itself or does it require independent treatment? Patients may require psychotherapeutic interventions such as cognitive behavioural therapy and families may need to be involved if there are problems in relationships. There are particular issues regarding the maintenance of the morale of patients in the long term [17].

Some patients will require antidepressant medication; most psychiatrists would use an antidepressant to treat a depressed patient with schizophrenia sooner or later. A recent trial of sertraline (a specific serotonin reuptake inhibitor [SSRI]) versus imipramine (a tricyclic antidepressant) in patients with postpsychotic depressive disorder showed the two drugs to be equally effective. The SSRI was, however, significantly advantageous in terms of rapid onset of action; it also had less side effects and reduced the risk of schizophrenic relapse [18]. In general, the combination of conventional antipsychotic drugs and antidepressant drugs may be helpful, although benefits may be quite limited [19]. The evidence for co-medication with anticonvulsants and lithium is less persuasive.

There is growing opinion that most, if not all, atypical antipsychotic drugs may produce an antidepressant effect in schizophrenia [20,21]. This is predicated on their serotonergic, alpha-adrenergic and muscarinic properties, actions that are thought to be intrinsically antidepressant in nature. Most of a relatively small number of studies demonstrate superiority to placebo, conventional antipsychotic drugs, or both, regarding depressive symptoms.

As mentioned above, there is an overlap between depression and dysphoria (the latter being part of the neuroleptic-induced deficit syndrome), for example, subjective feelings of general malaise, 'feeling drugged up like a zombie' etc. It should be possible to distinguish neuroleptic-induced dysphoria from a genuine depressive syndrome on phenomenological grounds. Some authors take the view that dysphoria is a subtle form of akathisia [15]. Certainly, dysphoria is one of the side effects most frequently complained of by patients [22]. Two placebo-controlled studies have demonstrated that classical antipsychotic drugs, at least in reasonably small doses in stable patients, do not appear to cause depressive symptoms [23,24], but this does not rule out the induction of dysphoria. Again, the 'rule of thumb' is to use a well-tolerated treatment at the minimum effective dose.

Premorbid personality

Many patients have a history of prominent 'schizoid' traits of social inactivity, difficulty expressing emotion, eccentricity etc. A full history from an informant will give an indication of how much of the presentation is long standing as opposed to how much is new. The deterioration of pre-existing personality traits is a well-recognised phenomenon across the spectrum of mental illness. It is likely that 'schizoid' traits do increase the risk of developing negative symptoms, perhaps even representing a subclinical manifestation of schizophrenia. Whether these traits are less likely to be modified by psychiatric treatment than negative symptoms in patients with an apparently normal premorbid personality is unknown; there is no literature to be found on this question. Even so, attempts at treatment, particularly in the form of rehabilitation, are worth trying.

Institutional environment

Asylums are not the only places where patients may live an impoverished existence, with few stimuli to which to respond. Patients may be quietly institutionalized in their family homes or in care homes and there may be an understandable reluctance on the part of their relatives and carers to 'rock the boat' by introducing new drugs, psychotherapies and activities. A gentle rehabilitative approach with the emphasis on enriching the environment and experience of the patient would appear to make sense in these circumstances. It may be necessary to involve the family or carers by helping them understand why there is room for improvement and how this can be brought about, and trying to help them adjust to new situations along the way (eg, unaccustomed assertiveness on the part of the patient).

References

1. Flaum M, Andreasen N. **The reliability of distinguishing primary versus secondary negative symptoms.** *Compr Psychiatry* 1995; **36**:421–427.
2. Overall JE, Gorham DR. **The brief psychiatric rating scale.** *Psychol Rep* 1962; **10**:799–812.
3. Krawiecka M, Goldberg D, Vaughan M. **A standardized psychiatric assessment scale for rating chronic psychotic patients.** *Acta Psychiatr Scand* 1977; **55**:299–308.
4. Hyde CE. **The Manchester Scale. A standardised psychiatric assessment for rating chronic psychotic patients.** *Br J Psychiatry Suppl* 1989; **155**:45–48.
5. Mortimer AM, Lund CE, McKenna PJ et al. **Rating of negative symptoms using the High Royds Evaluation of Negativity (HEN) Scale.** *Br J Psychiatry Suppl* 1989; **160**:89–92.
6. Andreasen NC. *The Comprehensive Assessment of Symptoms and History.* Iowa City: The University of Iowa College of Medicine, 1987.
7. Kay SR, Opler LA, Lindenmayer JP. **The Positive and Negative Syndrome Scale (PANSS): rationale and standardisation.** *Br J Psychiatry Suppl* 1989; **155**:59–67.
8. Moller HJ, van Praag HM, Aufdembrinke B et al. **Negative symptoms in schizophrenia: considerations for clinical trials. Working group on negative symptoms in schizophrenia.** *Psychopharmacology (Berl)* 1994; **115**:221–228.
9. Casey DE. **Clozapine: neuroleptic-induced EPS and tardive dyskinesia.** *Psychopharmacology (Berl)* 1989; **99**(Suppl):S47–S53.
10. Allan ER, Sison CE, Alpert M et al. **The relationship between negative symptoms of schizophrenia and extrapyramidal side effects with haloperidol and olanzapine.** *Psychopharmacol Bull* 1998; **34**:71–74.
11. Johnstone EC, Crow TJ, Ferrier IN et al. **Adverse effects of anticholinergic medication on positive schizophrenic symptoms.** *Psychol Med* 1983; **13**:513–527.
12. Singh MM, Kay SR, Opler LA. **Anticholinergic-neuroleptic antagonism in terms of positive and negative symptoms of schizophrenia: implications for psychobiological subtyping.** *Psychol Med* 1987; **17**:39–48.
13. Anonymous. **Prophylactic use of anticholinergics in patients on long-term neuroleptic treatment. A consensus statement. World Health Organization heads of centres collaborating in WHO co-ordinated studies on biological aspects of mental illness.** *Br J Psychiatry* 1990, **156**:412.
14. Lader M. **Neuroleptic-induced deficit syndrome: old problem, new challenge.** *J Psychopharmacol* 1993; **7**:392–393.
15. Barnes TR, McPhillips MA. **How to distinguish between the neuroleptic-induced deficit syndrome, depression and disease-related negative symptoms in schizophrenia.** *Int Clin Psychopharmacol* 1995; **10**(Suppl 3):115–121.
16. Lewander T. **Neuroleptics and the neuroleptic-induced deficit syndrome.** *Acta Psychiatr Scand* Suppl 1994; **380**:8–13.
17. Weiden PJ. **Psychosocial treatment of depression in schizophrenia.** In: *Managing the Depressive Symptoms of Schizophrenia.* Edited by PEJ Keck. London: Science Press, 1999;58–72.
18. Kirli S, Caliskan M. **A comparative study of sertraline versus imipramine in postpsychotic depressive disorder of schizophrenia.** *Schizophr Res* 1998; **33**:103–111.
19. Sernyak MJ, Petrakis IL. **Pharmacological treatment strategies: antidepressant and typical antipsychotic agents.** In: *Managing the Depressive Symptoms of Schizophrenia.* Edited by PEJ Keck. London: Science Press, 1999;30–43.
20. Anonymous. **Atypical antipsychotics for treatment of depression in schizophrenia and affective disorders. Collaborative Working Group on Clinical Trial Evaluations.** *J Clin Psychiatry* 1998; **59**(Suppl 12):41–45.
21. Keck PEJ. **Pharmacological treatment strategies: atypical antipsychotics.** In: *Managing the Depressive Symptoms of Schizophrenia.* Edited by PEJ Keck. London: Science Press, 1999;44–72.
22. Gerlach J, Larsen EB. **Subjective experience and mental side-effects of antipsychotic treatment.** *Acta Psychiatr Scand Suppl* 1999; **395**:113–117.
23. Wistedt B, Palmstierna T. **Depressive symptoms in chronic schizophrenic patients after withdrawal of long-acting neuroleptics.** *J Clin Psychiatry* 1983; **44**:369–371.
24. Hogarty GE, Munetz MR. **Pharmacogenic depression among outpatient schizophrenic patients: a failure to substantiate.** *J Clin Psychopharmacol* 1984; **4**:17–24.

Chapter 7

Pharmacological treatment approaches

General philosophy

It is recommended that negative symptoms be addressed as early as possible, because of the accepted difficulty in treating established primary negative syndromes. This means during the prodrome of the illness if this can be detected (eg, through surveillance of high-risk groups) and certainly during and after the first episode. The findings that negative symptoms may precede positive symptoms prodromally [1], and that the negative picture is quite fluid during the first episode and afterwards [2], provide a further rationale for early intervention before the deficit state is established.

All conventional neuroleptic drugs are strong dopamine receptor blockers and this is thought to represent their mechanism of action in the treatment of positive symptoms. In theory, therefore, conventional neuroleptic drugs should not be effective for negative symptoms and may even worsen them; there is evidence to support this (*see* Chapter 4). Dose reduction of conventional neuroleptic drugs may be tried if the dose is particularly high, as this may relieve Parkinsonism without compromising positive symptom control. It has been demonstrated, however, that establishing a low serum level of the neuroleptic drug will only reduce negative symptoms that were mild in the first place; there is no improvement in severe symptoms [3] and the risk of a relapse of positive symptoms should always be considered. There is, therefore, no evidence that low-dose conventional neuroleptic drugs are indicated for the treatment of problematic primary negative symptoms.

The other important effect of neuroleptic drugs is the prevention of relapse. Because the negative syndrome tends to be associated with long periods of inadequate treatment, both before diagnosis and in the context of repeated relapses, it is reasonable to assume that prevention of the development of the negative syndrome is possible via good clinical management of compliance. This needs to be addressed, ideally, at the first episode, with the patient and family undergoing a process of education and counselling that stresses the meaning of the diagnosis, the mechanisms of coping with the illness and resulting stresses, and the importance of continuing the recommended treatment. There is increasing opinion that one of the atypical antipsychotic drugs should be prescribed to the first-episode patient because of their mild side effect profiles and possibly superior antipsychotic efficacy.

Differentiation between direct and indirect effects of neuroleptic drugs on negative symptoms

There has been much argument in the literature regarding the extent to which neuroleptic drugs reduce primary negative symptoms [4]. Clearly, neuroleptic drugs may control positive symptoms and depression, while newer drugs may reduce previously existing EPS. This may relieve pseudonegative symptoms without any genuine impact on the primary symptoms. This issue is important, because it is good clinical practice to determine the origin of negative symptoms and treat them appropriately. Antidepressants and psychological therapies may be appropriate for depression; psychosocial interventions or adjunctive treatments may reduce uncontrolled positive symptoms; and reduction of the neuroleptic drug dose alone may resolve side effects. It is, therefore, misleading and unhelpful to claim that a drug is efficacious in the negative syndrome unless this is demonstrable for primary negative symptoms. There are, however, considerable methodological difficulties in demonstrating such efficacy directly [4].

One solution is path analysis [5,6], a statistical technique that allows the estimation of the degree to which the effect of a neuroleptic drug on negative symptoms is mediated by its effects on other symptoms. Certain causal relationships are assumed and other assumptions concern: the linearity of relationships between other symptoms and negative symptoms; the inclusion of all relevant variables in the model; and the independence of predictor variables. Data from a study comparing risperidone with haloperidol have been fitted to this model [7]. Depression was not included since the authors found no association between depression and negative symptoms. Baseline values of the variables themselves were significant predictors of their degree of change. The estimates of direct and indirect effects of treatment on negative symptoms demonstrated a direct effect of risperidone, but not haloperidol. This is equivalent to saying that effects on positive symptoms or EPS do not mediate the risperidone effect on negative symptoms, therefore, it must be a specific effect on primary symptoms. The authors concluded, however, that the effect demonstrated had no established relevance to clinical therapeutic effects.

Atypical neuroleptic drugs and negative symptoms

In animal studies, atypical antipsychotic drugs display a bewildering range of neurotransmitter receptor affinities. All atypical antipsychotic drugs have, however, higher affinity for 5-HT-2A receptors than dopamine-2 receptors [8]. This is their sole common point of difference from conventional antipsychotic drugs (except amisulpride) and is of considerable interest, since there is good evidence that 5-HT-2A-receptor antagonism is associated with therapeutic effects on negative symptoms [9,10]. Atypical antipsychotic drugs may be divided into three groups: those with significant receptor affinity in addition to that for dopamine-2 and 5-HT-2A receptors (clozapine, olanzapine, quetiapine and zotepine); those with significant affinities limited to dopamine-2 and 5-HT-2A receptors (risperidone and ziprasidone); and those that selectively bind to dopamine-3 receptors (sulpiride and amisulpride).

Amisulpride

Amisulpride selectively binds to dopamine-2 and dopamine-3 receptors in animal models. There is some limbic selectivity (ie, the striatum is relatively spared), which should avoid Parkinsonian side effects to some degree. Some of the dopamine receptors are presynaptic autoreceptors, antagonism of which tends to increase dopaminergic neurotransmission. As predicted, there are some positive effects on animal models of negative symptoms [11]. These include increasing regional glucose use (a proxy for neuronal activity) in the rat equivalent of human brain areas involved in cognition, motivation and emotion [12].

In a large, double-blind, randomized trial [13] that met criteria for valid evaluation [19], amisulpride in low doses (100 mg/day) was compared with placebo. Patients had high levels of negative symptoms and a Diagnostic and Statistical Manual, revised third edition (DSMIII-R) diagnosis of residual schizophrenia. There were substantial decreases in negative symptoms of approximately one-third in the amisulpride group, and EPS were at placebo levels. Positive, depressive and general symptoms were also significantly reduced, but the absolute changes were far less in percentage terms. Dropout rates were 20% for the active treatment group and 40% for the placebo group. It is difficult to find serious fault with this study or its findings, except to say that an active (conventional) comparator, had it produced an efficacy equivalent to placebo, would have made arguments for switching 'deficit' patients to low-dose amisulpride difficult to refute.

Two other studies of similar patients, although methodologically not as strong, reported comparable findings [14,15]. A one-year study of long-term inpatients with chronic schizophrenia (selected for predominant negative symptoms) compared low-dose amisulpride with haloperidol [16]. The study found no significant improvements with either drug, but there were trends in favour of amisulpride. Patients on haloperidol required significantly more anticholinergic medication. This result may be a function of the patient sample, in which the negative symptoms were longstanding and relatively resistant to treatment with amisulpride. If this is the case, it emphasises the need to deal with negative symptoms effectively before they become ingrained.

Clozapine

Clozapine has weak affinity for dopamine-2 receptors and strong affinity for serotonin 5-HT-2A receptors. It has significant affinities for histaminergic, adrenergic, cholinergic and dopamine-4 receptors, but the therapeutic importance of these affinities is not clear except in terms of side effects such as sedation and hypotension. EPS are conspicuous by their absence. The use of clozapine is limited to treatment-resistant patients (the definition of which often includes a negative syndrome) owing to its side effect of neutropenia, which occurs in one in 43 patients and which necessitates regular blood counts. After the first year of treatment with clozapine, however, there is no evidence that neutropenia develops more frequently than with conventional neuroleptic treatment.

The therapeutic actions of clozapine are poorly understood. In studies of monkeys, clozapine abolished amphetamine-induced social isolation [17], a paradigm that is thought to model negative symptoms and that is unaffected by conventional antipsychotic drugs. The neurochemistry is believed to involve antagonism of the dopamine-1 receptor, for which clozapine has some affinity. In a study comparing early-onset patients established on clozapine with similar patients on conventional drugs, there were significantly higher blood levels of serotonin, noradrenaline and their metabolites; serotonin levels were inversely related to negative symptoms, and levels of the noradrenaline metabolite MHPG were inversely related to depression [18]. These findings were replicated in treatment-resistant patients commenced on clozapine compared with patients remaining on 'treatment as usual'. The increases in noradrenaline and MHPG tended to be limited to clozapine responders, as were inverse associations between negative symptoms, blood serotonin and noradrenaline levels. The authors suggested that baseline adrenaline levels predicted response to clozapine.

In animal models, clozapine is able to increase expression of the immediate early gene *c-fos* in cortical limbic and prefrontal regions; this is thought to be a marker of dopamine release in these areas. Conventional neuroleptic drugs, such as haloperidol, show this effect more in striatal areas. When there are induced lesions in infralimbic prefrontal areas, the ability of clozapine to induce *c-fos* is actually enhanced [19]. Given the putative frontal pathophysiology and decreased dopaminergic activity in patients with negative symptoms, this finding may be relevant to the therapeutic impact of clozapine on negative symptoms.

There seems little doubt that clozapine is superior to conventional treatment for negative symptoms [20–23]; only one early study argues for equivalence [24]. The longer the period of study, the greater the effect seen. It is well known that clozapine, in contrast to accepted wisdom regarding all other antipsychotic drugs, may continue to improve patients over months or even years. The sheer volume of this work, the degree of change and the experience of clinicians perhaps outweigh the fact that most of these studies do no meet the consensus criteria [25]. Argument remains as to whether primary symptoms, pseudonegative symptoms or both are relieved, most studies being methodologically incapable of teasing this out. Improvement does not, however, depend on high levels of negative symptoms to begin with [26] and can occur even if other aspects of psychopathology remain the same [27].

Clozapine remains the treatment of choice for treatment-resistant patients, but for patients with relatively isolated negative symptoms it may be worth trying an alternative atypical drug first for six weeks.

Olanzapine

The affinities of olanzapine are similar to those of clozapine, but olanzapine blocks dopamine-2 more strongly. EPS are reported at placebo level within the dosage range;

sedation and weight gain (particularly) may cause problems. Four randomized, double-blind, controlled studies have assessed the effects of olanzapine on negative symptoms. The first study showed that olanzapine was superior to placebo [28]. The second showed that olanzapine was superior to placebo and haloperidol [29]. In the third, there was a trend towards superiority of olanzapine over haloperidol [30] and in the fourth, once again, significant superiority of olanzapine over haloperidol [31]. Data from the second study were subject to path analysis, which suggested that the effects of haloperidol on negative symptoms were almost entirely accounted for by its effects on positive symptoms (hence, it modified pseudonegative symptoms), and this was offset by its increasing EPS. By contrast, the relief of pseudonegativity [32] accounted for only 20% of the effect of olanzapine.

The greatest mean change in negative symptoms occurred in the second and third studies; with olanzapine given at 15 mg/day, there was a substantial reduction of approximately one-third in rating scale scores. A small open study of treatment-resistant patients also demonstrated significant improvements in negative symptoms [33]. Olanzapine is, thus, a logical choice as a first alternative for patients on conventional treatment with prominent negative symptoms, particularly those with EPS. Weight gain and risk of development of type 2 diabetes mellitus are, however, increasing sources of concern and warrant consideration prior to treatment.

Quetiapine
Quetiapine, like clozapine, is effective in the monkey social isolation model of negative symptoms [34] and does have some affinity for dopamine-1 receptors. Quetiapine has a broad receptor binding profile, however, with high affinity for dopamine-2 and dopamine-1 receptors. EPS occur at placebo levels across the dosage range. In view of this, it is surprising that several studies have failed to demonstrate better efficacy than conventional treatment for negative symptoms [34], although quetiapine is significantly better than placebo. One study of quetiapine versus chlorpromazine in patients with acute exacerbation of subchronic or chronic schizophrenia or schizophreniform disorder demonstrated a trend towards superiority for quetiapine, but this did not reach statistical significance [35]. In a recent meta-analysis of studies, which demonstrated that olanzapine and risperidone were more effective than haloperidol, quetiapine was actually less effective. Therefore, quetiapine would not necessarily offer a first choice alternative for patients on conventional treatment with isolated problematic or unresolved negative symptoms.

Risperidone
Risperidone has a high affinity for 5-HT-2A receptors, which it acts upon preferentially in the medial prefrontal cortex [36]. The dopamine-2 receptor affinity of risperidone is weaker and more generalized. EPS of risperidone are dose related, but much less than with conventional drugs; in groups of patients on 6 mg/day or

less (recommended therapeutic dose is 4–8 mg), the incidence is no more than placebo. The evidence for superiority over conventional antipsychotic drugs in the treatment of negative symptoms is mixed; most studies do not accord with consensus methodology. Some studies found a beneficial effect that was not greater than the effect of a comparator, leading to suggestions that differences in EPS were related to pseudonegative symptom differences [7,37,38]. Despite these reservations, two further analyses using different methodologies support a direct component to the effect of risperidone on negative symptoms [5,39]. Even so, changes in PANSS rating totals were at most five points, a finding of uncertain significance considering that the scale range is up to 42 points. A study by the authors (Mortimer *et al.*, in preparation), which did attempt to meet consensus criteria, found that positive, negative and depressive symptoms all improved significantly with risperidone treatment and by about the same, moderate amount; the major finding was a halving of EPS levels.

Three meta-analyses cast further light on the matter of risperidone and negative symptoms. In one study of 11 randomized controlled trials, the difference in PANSS negative scores between risperidone and conventional treatment was almost statistically significant [40]. A second study of six trials demonstrated a significantly higher response rate for negative symptoms (20% or greater reduction in ratings); 43% more patients were responders to risperidone than to haloperidol [41]. A third meta-analysis of five studies reported 60% greater efficacy for negative symptoms than conventional treatment [42].

One study found the negative symptom levels to be closely associated with performance on an executive test, both before and after treatment with risperidone [43]. Although there was no comparator drug or test, this indirectly supports an effect of risperidone on primary negative symptoms; the assumption is made that both this type of cognition and negative symptoms have a common substrate, which is acted upon by risperidone.

Overall, it would seem that risperidone is well worth trying in patients with negative symptoms who do not respond to conventional treatment, and the symptoms treated may include primary as well as pseudonegative symptoms. Patients who are not prone to EPS and/or who are prone to oversedation or weight gain would be particularly suitable for risperidone instead of olanzapine or zotepine.

Sulpiride

There is no evidence that sulpiride, a selective dopamine-2- and dopamine-3-receptor blocker, has a better effect on negative symptoms than conventional neuroleptic drugs. It has, however, a mild side effect profile and is said to be antidepressant when given at low doses, which should help to avoid the pseudonegative syndromes resulting from EPS and depression of mood.

Ziprasidone

The most important affinities of ziprasidone are for dopamine-2 and several serotonin receptors, including 5-HT-2A receptors [44]. Ziprasidone appears to have EPS at placebo levels. There is as yet no evidence of better efficacy for negative symptoms compared with conventional treatment [45], although it is better than placebo. Ziprasidone is also better than placebo for depressive symptoms [46], but further trial results are awaited.

Zotepine

Zotepine binds to numerous receptors, with particular affinity for dopamine-1 and dopamine-2 receptors. The incidence of EPS is much less than with conventional antipsychotic drugs. The first randomized controlled studies reported equal efficacy to conventional treatment for negative symptoms [47–49]; a later study of patients with residual schizophrenia and high levels of negative symptoms [50] found zotepine to be superior to haloperidol, with 24% as opposed to 14% reduction in symptom levels. This was confirmed by a further comparison in chronic patients [51]. One study even showed zotepine to be equivalent to clozapine in decreasing negative symptoms [52]. The manufacturer's product monograph [53] presents a meta-analysis of negative efficacy measures from some of these studies, plus several others 'on file'. Overall, zotepine was shown to be superior to placebo or active comparator in all studies, with a maximum difference between groups of up to half a standard deviation. Therefore, zotepine is worth trying in patients with negative symptoms who do not respond to conventional treatment, although currently there is little evidence for a direct effect on primary symptoms.

Other psychotropic drugs and negative symptoms

Antidepressants

Ideally, studies of the effects of antidepressants on negative symptoms should always use a measure of depressive symptoms in order to separate out pseudonegativity.

Tricyclic drugs

One of the side effects of tricyclic drugs is to reduce the sensitivity of inhibitory dopaminergic autoreceptors. This should result in increased dopaminergic neurotransmission with possibly an improvement in negative symptoms. Reviews of studies support a partial reduction on such treatment [54].

Serotonergic drugs

There is significant evidence that adding SSRI antidepressants to standard antipsychotic treatment improves negative symptoms of schizophrenia [10]. One study of patients with predominantly negative symptoms found an improvement with the SSRI fluvoxamine, but not with maprotiline (an antidepressant acting on noradrenergic neurotransmission). Depressive symptoms were low and did not change. It was concluded that fluvoxamine ameliorated negative symptoms through a serotonergic mechanism separate from any antidepressant effect [55].

A small study of eight patients with predominant negative or depressive symptoms reported that the antidepressant nefazodone (which blocks 5-HT-2A receptors) brought about reductions in negative symptoms of about one-third, with an even greater improvement in depressive symptoms of 60% [56]. Trazodone is a similar drug, which is much more sedating. In a larger placebo-controlled study, adding trazodone to stable neuroleptic treatment improved negative symptoms significantly (by 10–15%), but only three of 26 patients were rated as moderately clinically improved [57].

Cyproheptadine, which also blocks serotonin receptors, has been used to augment conventional neuroleptic drugs in a small double-blind, placebo-controlled study. In the study, there was a small, but significant, improvement in negative, but not positive, symptoms in the active medication group [58].

Monoamine oxidase inhibitors

MAOIs have a theoretical role in reducing negative symptoms because of their enhancement of noradrenergic and dopaminergic function. One small study suggests this to be the case in practice [59]. Augmentation with selegiline, a monoamine oxidase-B inhibitor, which selectively enhances dopaminergic activity, was found to benefit negative symptoms in a case series of three patients [60]. An open study of 21 patients with prominent negative symptoms produced impressive results, with a mean reduction of 35% in negative symptoms after six weeks; reductions in depressive symptoms and EPS were just as impressive, although positive symptoms were not exacerbated [61].

Nonbenzodiazepine hypnotic drugs

Substituting zopiclone, a nonbenzodiazepine hypnotic drug, for benzodiazepine in patients with schizophrenia has been shown to have beneficial effects on both sleep architecture and negative symptoms in one study [62].

Glutamatergic drugs

A small placebo-controlled study used glycine to potentiate NMDA-receptor-mediated neurotransmission in a group of patients with chronic schizophrenia. Negative symptoms improved in the glycine, but not the placebo, group [63]. In a small study of high-dose oral glycine, two of five patients reduced their negative symptoms by at least 20%; the improvement was related to blood glycine levels [64]. A more recent review has suggested that glycine, its prodrug milacemide and other glycinergic agents such as D-cycloserine may be useful [65]. A recent placebo-controlled crossover study of the addition of glycine to antipsychotic treatment reported an average fall of 30% of both negative and general symptoms in treatment-resistant patients; the improvement was unrelated to changes in EPS and depression. Furthermore, the clinical response was strongly associated with low pre-treatment serum levels of glycine [66]. In one small open-label study, where D-cycloserine, an anti-tuberculosis drug, was added to conventional neuroleptic treatment in patients selected for prominent negative symptoms, the negative symptoms improved by 21% and performance at a prefrontal task was significantly improved [67].

Sigma receptors are thought to modulate both glutamatergic and dopaminergic systems [68]. The theoretical advantage of sigma antagonists is their potential selectivity (ie, no unwanted direct dopaminergic effects); however, there has been only limited success so far in their applicability to the treatment of negative symptoms [69].

Dopaminergic agonists

Dopamine inhibitory autoreceptor agonists, such as roxindole, eventually produce postsynaptic receptor supersensitivity, which would be expected to reduce negative symptoms assuming the presence of adequate dopamine. Despite some positive findings with these drugs, overall, studies do not support effectiveness conclusively [54]. Dopamine-2-receptor agonists, such as levodopa and bromocriptine, and experimental partial agonists, may produce some improvements [39], but the induction of positive symptoms may be problematic, as when amphetamine is administered to patients. There would seem little point in administering such drugs in the presence of a conventional neuroleptic drug, which would simply compete for the dopamine-2-receptor site.

Psychotropic and other drugs ineffective against negative symptoms

Psychotropic and other drugs ineffective against negative symptoms include propranolol, clonidine and benzodiazepines. Anticholinergic drugs may appear to benefit negative symptoms, but this is inextricably confused with their motor effects and there is a tendency to exacerbate positive symptoms [70,71]. Lithium and carbamazepine enhance the antipsychotic effects of neuroleptic drugs in general, but there is no evidence for a disproportionate improvement in negative symptoms.

Figure 7.1 shows an algorithm for treating problematic negative symptoms.

Algorithm for treating problematic negative symptoms

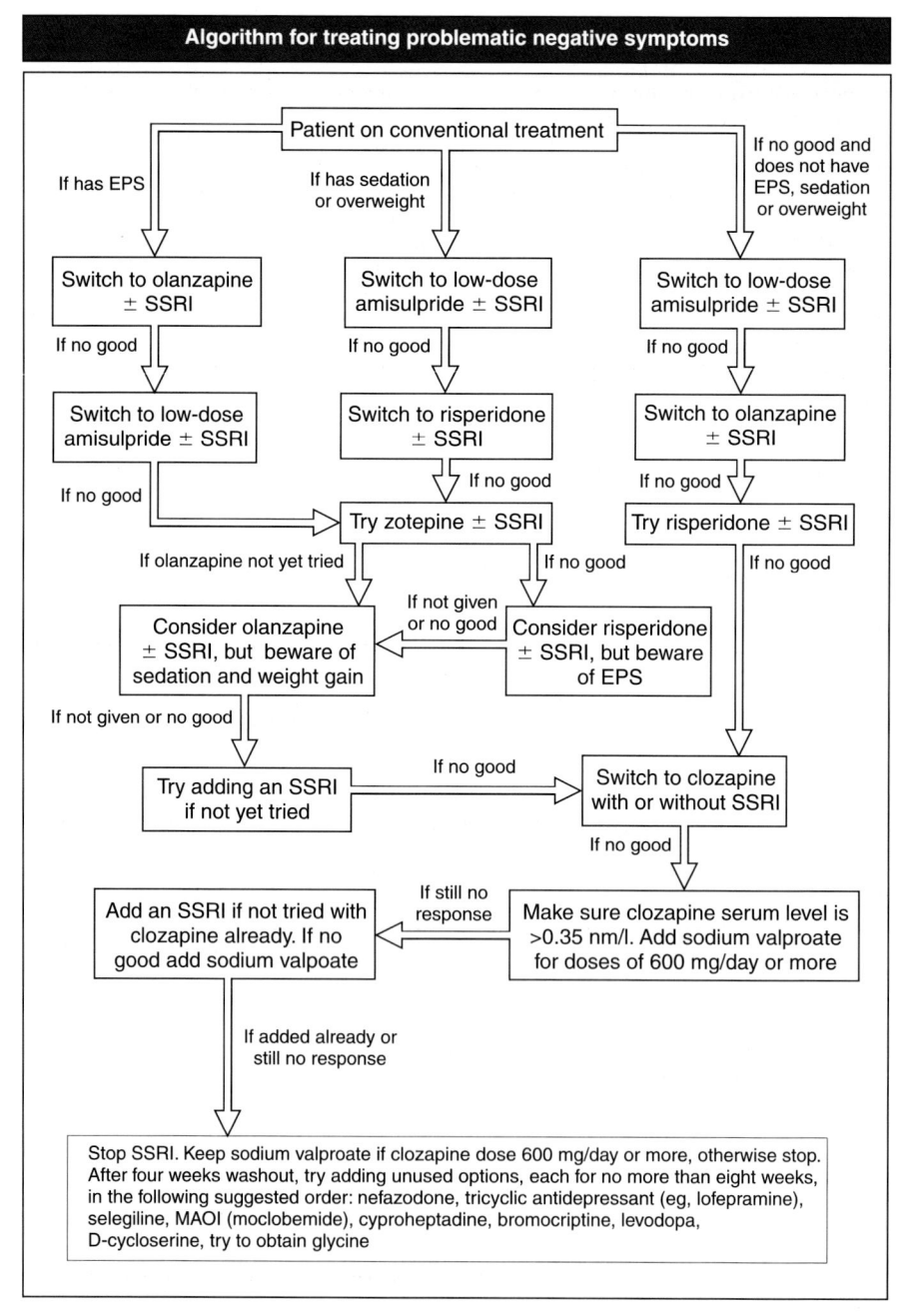

```
                    Patient on conventional treatment
                    ┌────────────┬────────────────┐
                    │            │                │
  If has EPS     If has sedation            If no good and
                 or overweight              does not have
                                            EPS, sedation
                                            or overweight
       ▼              ▼                         ▼
  Switch to      Switch to low-dose        Switch to low-dose
  olanzapine     amisulpride ± SSRI        amisulpride ± SSRI
  ± SSRI
  If no good     If no good                If no good
       ▼              ▼                         ▼
  Switch to low-dose   Switch to risperidone   Switch to olanzapine
  amisulpride ± SSRI   ± SSRI                  ± SSRI
  If no good                If no good         If no good
       ▼                         ▼                  ▼
                    Try zotepine ± SSRI     Try risperidone ± SSRI

  If olanzapine not yet tried   If no good   If no good
                    If not given
                    or no good
       ▼                              ▼
  Consider olanzapine         Consider risperidone
  ± SSRI, but beware of       ± SSRI, but beware
  sedation and weight gain    of EPS

  If not given or no good
       ▼                  If no good       ▼
  Try adding an SSRI ─────────────▶ Switch to clozapine
  if not yet tried                   with or without SSRI
                                     If no good
                                          ▼
                    If still no    Make sure clozapine serum level is
                    response       >0.35 nm/l. Add sodium valproate
  Add an SSRI if not tried with ◀──  for doses of 600 mg/day or more
  clozapine already. If no
  good add sodium valpoate

       If added already or
       still no response
              ▼
```

Stop SSRI. Keep sodium valproate if clozapine dose 600 mg/day or more, otherwise stop. After four weeks washout, try adding unused options, each for no more than eight weeks, in the following suggested order: nefazodone, tricyclic antidepressant (eg, lofepramine), selegiline, MAOI (moclobemide), cyproheptadine, bromocriptine, levodopa, D-cycloserine, try to obtain glycine

Figure 7.1. EPS, extrapyramidal side effects; SSRI, selective serotonin re-uptake inhibitor; MAOI, monoamine oxidase inhibitor.

References

1. Hafner H, Maurer K. **Are there two types of schizophrenia? True onset and sequence of positive and negative syndromes prior to first admission.** In: *Negative versus Positive Schizophrenia.* Edited by A Maneros, NC Andreasen and MT Tsuang. New York: Springer, 1992;134–160.
2. Edwards J, McGorry PD, Waddell FM et al. **Enduring negative symptoms in first-episode psychosis: comparison of six methods using follow-up data.** *Schizophr Res* 1999; **40**:147–158.
3. Volavka J, Cooper TB, Czobor P et al. **Effects of varying haloperidol plasma levels on negative symptoms in schizophrenia and schizoaffective disorder.** *Psychopharmacol Bull* 1996; **32**:75–79.
4. Moller HJ. **Neuroleptic treatment of negative symptoms in schizophrenic patients. Efficacy problems and methodology difficulties.** *Eur Neuropsychopharmacol* 1993; **3**:3–11.
5. Moller HJ, Muller H, Borison RL et al. **A path-analytical approach to differentiate between direct and indirect drug effects on negative symptoms in schizophrenic patients. A re-evaluation of the North American risperidone study.** *Eur Arch Psychiatry Clin Neurosci* 1995; **245**:45–49.
6. Moller HJ, Muller H. **Statistical differentiation between direct and indirect effects of neuroleptics on negative symptoms.** *Eur Arch Psychiatry Clin Neurosci* 1997; **247**:1–5.
7. Marder SR, Meibach RC. **Risperidone in the treatment of schizophrenia.** *Am J Psychiatry* 1994; **151**:825–835.
8. Schotte A, Janssen PF, Gommeren W et al. **Risperidone compared with new and reference antipsychotic drugs: in vitro and in vivo receptor binding.** *Psychopharmacology (Berl)* 1996; **124**:57–73.
9. Schmidt CJ, Sorensen SM, Kefine JH et al. **The role of 5-HT2A receptors in antipsychotic activity.** *Life Sci* 1995; **56**:2209–2222.
10. Leysen JE, Gommeren W, Schotte A. **Serotonin receptor subtypes: possible roles and implications in antipsychotic drug action.** In: *Serotonin in Antipsychotic Treatment.* Edited by JM Kane, H Moller and F Awouters. New York: Marcel Dekker, 1996;51–75.
11. Scatton B, Claustre Y, Cudennec A et al. **Amisulpride: from animal pharmacology to therapeutic action.** *Int Clin Psychopharmacol* 1997; **12**(Suppl. 2):S29–S36.
12. Cudennec A, Fage D, Benavides J et al. **Effects of amisulpride, an atypical antipsychotic which blocks preferentially presynaptic dopamine autoreceptors, on integrated functional cerebral activity in the rat.** *Brain Res* 1997; **768**:257–265.
13. Danion JM, Rein W, Fleurot O. **Improvement of schizophrenic patients with primary negative symptoms treated with amisulpride. Amisulpride Study Group.** *Am J Psychiatry* 1999; **156**:610–616.
14. Boyer P, Lecrubier Y, Peuch AJ et al. **Treatment of negative symptoms in schizophrenia with amisulpride.** *Br J Psychiatry* 1995; **166**:68–72.
15. Loo H, Poirier-Littre MF, Theron M et al. **Amisulpride versus placebo in the medium-term treatment of the negative symptoms of schizophrenia.** *Br J Psychiatry* 1997; **170**:18–22.
16. Speller JC, Barnes TR, Curson DA et al. **One-year, low-dose neuroleptic study of in-patients with chronic schizophrenia characterised by persistent negative symptoms. Amisulpride v. haloperidol.** *Br J Psychiatry* 1997; **171**:564–568.
17. Ellenbroek BA, Lubbers LJ, Cools AR. **Activity of 'seroquel' (ICI 204,636) in animal models for atypical properties of antipsychotics: a comparison with clozapine.** *Neuropsychopharmacology* 1996; **15**:406–416.
18. Schulz E, Fleischhacker C, Clement HW et al. **Blood biogenic amines during clozapine treatment of early-onset schizophrenia.** *J Neural Trans* 1997; **104**:1077–1089.
19. Roe DL, Bardgett ME, Csernansky CA et al. **Induction of Fos protein by anitpsychotic drugs in rat brain following kainic acid-induced limbic-cortical neuronal loss.** *Psychopharmacology (Berl)* 1998; **138**:151–158.
20. Kane J, Honigfeld G, Singer J et al. **Clozapine for the treatment-resistant schizophrenic. A double-blind comparison with chlorpromazine.** *Arch Gen Psychiatry* 1988; **45**:789–796.
21. Meltzer HY. **Dimensions of outcome with clozapine.** *Br J Psychiatry Suppl* 1992; **160**:46–53.
22. Lindenmayer JP, Grochowski S, Mabugat L. **Clozapine effects on positive and negative symptoms: a six-month trial in treatment-refractory schizophrenics.** *J Clin Psychopharmacol* 1994; **14**:201–204.
23. Breier A, Buchanan RW, Kirkpatrick B et al. **Effects of clonzapine on positive and negative symptoms in outpatients with schizophrenia.** *Am J Psychiatry* 1994; **151**:20–26.
24. Pickar D, Owen RR, Litman RE et al. **Clinical and biologic response to clozapine in patients with schizophrenia. Crossover comparison with fluphenazine.** *Arch Gen Psychiatry* 1992; **49**:345–353.

25. Moller HJ, van Praag HM, Aufdembrinke B et al. **Negative symptoms in schizophrenia: considerations for clinical trials. Working group on negative symptoms in schizophrenia.** *Psychopharmacology (Berl)* 1994; **115**:221–228.
26. Rosenheck R, Dunn L, Peszke M et al. **Impact of clozapine on negative symptoms and on the deficit syndrome in refractory schizophrenia. Department of Veterans Affairs Cooperative Study Group on Clozapine in Refractory Schizophrenia.** *Am J Psychiatry* 1999; **156**:88–93.
27. Brar JS, Chengappa KN, Parepally H et al. **The effects of clonzapine on negative symptoms in patients with schizophrenia with minimal positive symptoms.** *Ann Clin Psychiatry* 1997; **9**:227–234.
28. Beasley CM Jr, Sanger T, Satterlee W et al. **Olanzapine versus placebo: results of a double-blind, fixed-dose olanzapine trial.** *Psychopharmacology (Berl)* 1996; **124**:159–167.
29. Beasley CM Jr, Tollefson G, Tran P et al. **Olanzapine versus placebo and haloperidol: acute phase results of the North American double-blind olanzapine trial.** *Neuropsychopharmacology* 1996; **14**:111–123.
30. Beasley CM Jr, Hamilton SH, Crawford AM et al. **Olanzapine versus haloperidol: acute-phase results of the international double-blind olanzapine trial.** *Eur Neuropsychopharmacol* 1997; **7**:125–137.
31. Tollefson GD, Beaslet CM Jr, Tran PV et al. **Olanzapine versus haloperidol in the treatment of schizophrenia and schizoaffective and schizophreniform disorders: results of an international collaborative trial.** *Am J Psychiatry* 1997; **154**:457–465.
32. Tollefson GD, Sanger TM. **Negative symptoms: a path analytic approach to a double-blind, placebo- and haloperidol-controlled clinical trial with olanzapine.** *Am J Psychiatry* 1997; **154**:466–474.
33. Martin J, Gomez JC, Garcia-Bernando E et al. **Olanzapine in treatment-refractory schizophrenia: results of an open-label study. The Spanish Group for the Study of Olanzapine in Treatment-Refractory Schizophrenia.** *J Clin Psychiatry* 1997; **58**:479–483.
34. King DJ. **Drug treatment of the negative symptoms of schizophrenia.** *Eur Neuropsychopharmacol* 1998; **8**:33–42.
35. Peuskens J, Link CG. **A comparison of quetiapine and chlopromazine in the treatment of schizophrenia.** *Acta Psychiatr Scand* 1997; **96**:265–273.
36. Hertel P, Nomikos GG, Iurlo M et al. **Risperidone: regional effects in vivo on release and metabolism of dopamine and serotonin in the rat brain.** *Psychopharmacology (Berl)* 1996; **124**:74–86.
37. Chouinard G, Jones B, Remington G et al. **A Canadian multicenter placebo-controlled study of fixed doses of risperidone and haloperidol in the treatment of chronic schizophrenic patients.** *J Clin Psychopharmacol* 1993; **13**:25–40.
38. Schooler NR. **Negative symptoms in schizophrenia: assessment of the effect of risperidone.** *J Clin Psychiatry* 1994; **55**(Suppl.):22–28.
39. Lindenmayer JP. **New pharmacotherapeutic modalities for negative symptoms in psychosis.** *Acta Psychiatr Scand Suppl* 1995; **338**:15–19.
40. Song F. **Risperidone in the treatment of schizophrenia: a meta-analysis of randomized controlled trials.** *J Psychopharmacol* 1997; **11**:65–71.
41. Carman J, Peuskens J, Vangeneugden A. **Risperidone in the treatment of negative symptoms of schizophrenia: a meta-analysis.** *Int Clin Psychopharmacol* 1995; **10**:207–213.
42. Davis R, Janicak PG. **Risperidone: a new, novel (and better?) antipsychotic.** *Psychiatr Ann* 1996; **26**:78–87.
43. Rossi A, Mancini F, Stratta P et al. **Risperidone, negative symptoms and cognitive deficit in schizophrenia: an open study.** *Acta Psychiatr Scand* 1997; **95**:40–43.
44. Seeger TF, Seymour PA, Schmidt AW et al. **Ziprasidone (CP-88,059): a new antipsychotic with combined dopamine and serotonin receptor antagonist activity.** *J Pharmacol Exp Ther* 1995; **275**:101–113.
45. Gunn KP. **Ziprasidone: safety and efficacy.** *Schizophr Res* 1996; **18**:132–133.
46. Daniel DG, Zimbroff DL, Potkin SG et al. **Ziprasidone 80 mg/day and 160 mg/day in the acute exacerbation of schizophrenia and schizoaffective disorder: a 6-week placebo-controlled trial.** *Neuropsychopharmacology* 1999; **20**:491–505.
47. Fleischhacker WW, Barnas C, Stuppack C et al. **Zotepine vs. haloperidol in paranoid schizophrenia: a double-blind trial.** *Psychopharmacol Bull* 1989; **25**:97–100.
48. Muller-Spahn F, Dieterle DM, Ackenheil M. **[Clinical effectiveness of zotepine in the treatment of negative schizophrenic symptoms. Results of an open and a double-blind controlled trial.]** *Fortschr Neurol Psychiatr* 1991; **59**(Suppl. 1):30–35.
49. Dieterle DM, Muller-Spahn F, Ackenheil M. **[Effectiveness and tolerance of zotepine in a double-blind comparison with perazine in schizophrenic patients.]** *Fortschr Neurol Psychiatr* 1991; **59**(Suppl. 1):18–22.

50. Barnas C, Stuppack CH, Miller C et al. **Zotepine in the treatment of schizophrenic patients with prevailingly negative symptoms. A double-blind trial vs. haloperidol.** *Int Clin Psychopharmacol* 1992; 7:23–27.
51. Petit M, Raniwalla J, Tweed J et al. **A comparison of an atypical and typical antipsychotic, zotepine versus haloperidol in patients with acute exacerbation of schizophrenia: a parallel-group double-blind trial.** *Psychopharmacol Bull* 1996; 32:81–87.
52. Meyer-Lindenberg A, Gruppe H, Bauer U et al. **Improvement of cognitive function in schizophrenic patients receiving clozapine or zotepine: results from a double-blind study.** *Pharmacopsychiatry* 1997; 30:35–42.
53. Anonymous. *Zoleptil Product Monograph.* Complete Medical Communications International UK. 1999;26.
54. Rao ML, Moller HJ. **Biochemical findings of negative symptoms in schizophrenia and their putative relevance to pharmacologic treatment. A review.** *Neuropsychobiology* 1994; 30:160–172.
55. Silver H, Shmugliakov N. **Augmentation with fluvoxamine but not maprotiline improves negative symptoms in treated schizophrenia: evidence for a specific serotonergic effect from a double-blind study.** *J Clin Psychopharmacol* 1998; 18:208–211.
56. Joffe G, Appelberg B, Rimon R. **Adjunctive nefazodone in neuroleptic-treated schizophrenic patients with predominantly negative symptoms: an open prospective pilot study.** *Int Clin Psychopharmacol* 1999; 14:233–238.
57. Decina P, Mukherjee S, Bocola V et al. **Adjunctive trazodone in the treatment of negative symptoms of schizophrenia.** *Hosp Community Psychiatry* 1994; 45:1220–1223.
58. Akhondzadeh S, Mohammadi MR, Amini-Nooshabadi H et al. **Cyproheptadine in the treatment of chronic schizophrenia: a double-blind, placebo-controlled study.** *J Clin Pharm Ther* 1999; 24:49–52.
59. Bucci L. **The negative symptoms of schizophrenia and the monoamine oxidase inhibitors.** *Psychopharmacology (Berl)* 1987; 91:104–108.
60. Gupta S, Droney T, Kyser A et al. **Selegiline augmentation of antipsychotics for the treatment of negative symptoms in schizophrenia.** *Compr Psychiatry* 1999; 40:148–150.
61. Bodkin JA, Cohen BM, Salomon MS et al. **Treatment of negative symptoms in schizophrenia and schizoaffective disorder by selegiline augmentation of antipsychotic medication. A pilot study examining the role of dopamine.** *J Nerv Ment Dis* 1996; 184:295–301.
62. Kato M, Kajimura N, Okuma T et al. **Association between delta waves during sleep and negative symptoms in schizophrenia. Pharmaco-EEG studies using structurally different hypnotics.** *Neuropsychobiology* 1999; 39:165–172.
63. Javitt DC, Zylberman I, Zukin SR et al. **Amelioration of negative symptoms in schizophrenia by glycine.** *Am J Psychiatry* 1994; 151:1234–1236.
64. Leiderman E, Zylberman I, Zukin SR et al. **Preliminary investigation of high-dose oral glycine on serum levels and negative symptoms in schizophrenia: an open-label trial.** *Biol Psychiatry* 1996; 39:213–215.
65. Semba J. **[Glycine therapy of schizophrenia; its rationale and a review of clinical trials.]** *Nihon Shinkei Seishin Yakurigaku Zasshi* 1998; 18:71–80.
66. Heresco-Levy U, Javitt DC, Ermilov M et al. **Efficacy of high-dose glycine in the treatment of enduring negative symptoms of schizophrenia.** *Arch Gen Psychiatry* 1999; 56:29–36.
67. Goff DC, Tsai G, Manoach DS et al. **Dose-finding trial of D-cycloserine added to neuroleptics for negative symptoms in schizophrenia.** *Am J Psychiatry* 1995; 152:1213–1215.
68. Shim SS, Grant ER, Singh S et al. **Actions of butyrophenones and other antipsychotic agents at NMDA receptors: relationship with clinical effects and structural consideration.** *Neurochem Int* 1999; 34:167–175.
69. Modell S, Naber D, Holzbach R. **Efficacy and safety of an opiate sigma-receptor antagonist (SL 82.0715) in schizophrenic patients with negative symptoms: an open dose-range study.** *Pharmacopsychiatry* 1996; 29:63–66.
70. Johnstone EC, Crow TJ, Ferrier IN et al. **Adverse effects of anticholinergic medication on positive schizophrenic symptoms.** *Psychol Med* 1983; 13:513–527.
71. Singh MM, Kay SR, Opler LA. **Anticholinergic-neuroleptic antagonism in terms of positive and negative symptoms of schizophrenia: implications for psychobiological subtyping.** *Psychol Med* 1987; 17:39–48.

Chapter 8

Social and family approaches

Antipsychotic medication is generally considered mandatory in schizophrenia, not just to resolve positive symptoms, but perhaps more importantly to prevent relapse, and with it the development of chronic residual negative symptoms. Although antipsychotic drugs are necessary, they are, however, insufficient on their own to treat all aspects of the problems of patients and their families. A range of social and family approaches is essential to optimize the progress and well-being of the patient. This approach should include education for the patient and family about the illness; helping the patient and family accept the illness and adjust to the limitations it imposes; compliance counselling; problem solving for families with a mentally ill member; the detection of deterioration; effective use of services; and cognitive behavioural therapy for positive symptoms. These 'psychosocial interventions' should be, but rarely are, offered to all first-episode patients alongside pharmacological management.

Regarding patients with established negative symptoms, rehabilitation is the mainstay of treatment. This should not, however, preclude offering psychosocial interventions as appropriate ('better late than never'). 'Social skills training' is a particular form of rehabilitation that has been studied in the context of patients with negative symptoms.

Psychosocial interventions

Relatives and other carers need to be given frank information about negative symptoms and their implications. With an established syndrome that has been unresponsive to drug and rehabilitative approaches, expectations of the patient's capacity to achieve must be lowered. Difficulties arise when a relative refuses to accept the realities of loss of function, when painful feelings of anger and grief remain unexpressed and when no adjustments are made to accommodate the situation of the patient. Such problems may present as the following.

- A hostile or infantilizing attitude to the patient.
- A claustrophobic family atmosphere with over-involvement in the minutiae of the activities of the patient.
- Relatives and patient are together all the time, without a break for either.
- Helpless inability to cope.
- Angry demands that something be done without the inclination or ability to act on professional advice.

Such environments, containing relatives classically described as 'expressing high levels of emotion towards the patient', have been repeatedly associated with higher rates of relapse. Interventions such as social skills training, family psychoeducation and interpersonal problem solving training can lower levels of expressed emotion and reduce relapse rates substantially. There is no evidence that patients with predominant negative symptoms are more likely to have relatives in the high expressed emotion category, but given that families may find negative symptoms more of a burden than positive symptoms [1], perhaps there should be more awareness of a potential problem in this direction.

A grief counselling approach may be useful in working with families, in that relatives are encouraged to mourn the loss of the former function and future potential of the patient so that some adaptation can take place. Relief care (day care or respite periods) through a statutory or voluntary agency can also help the morale of the relatives and gives them and the patient a break from each other. Self-help groups organized locally or through one of the schizophrenia or mental health charities (National Schizophrenia Fellowship, Making Space, SANE, MIND etc; *see* Appendix VII) can assist relatives by providing support and breaking down feelings of isolation. It is essential to meet the inevitable 'search after meaning' of the family with reassurances that the patient's illness is not their fault.

An exploratory study of the strategies employed by both patients and relatives to cope with negative symptoms demonstrated clear benefits for those with more knowledge about schizophrenia. The patients and relatives used more strategies of different kinds so were more flexible and versatile and they reported higher levels of coping efficacy [2]. Perceived coping efficacy was highest for apathy and lowest for affective blunting.

Rehabilitation

The loss of self-care, communication and community skills that results from the negative syndrome is germane to the loss of independence and increased resource uptake in schizophrenia. Rehabilitation has much to offer during and after the optimization of pharmacological management; eventually rehabilitation should be continued in the community. At the simplest level, skills that are lacking are identified and attempts made to motivate the patient so that they can learn these skills again through repeated practice. Patients may need extra aids, such as printed instructions about the stages of cooking a meal or using a washing machine. It is important that the patient appreciates why such activities are useful and receives verbal and social reinforcement for improved performance. A behavioural programme may be set up in which the patient is rewarded for getting up, having a bath, doing laundry etc. Social skills training, the use of role play and opportunities to interact with the community outside the hospital, hostel or home, are all useful ways of helping the patient function better and the team to monitor progress. Outside contacts with family, friends or volunteers should always be encouraged. Sheltered work may help patients raise their self-esteem by achieving something, but exploitation should be guarded against. As an overall aim, the patient should spend more time on meaningful activities and less time doing nothing. Excessive time spent watching television or smoking, for example, should also be discouraged.

For patients unwilling to learn necessary skills, alternatives should be considered; the attitudes and values of people without schizophrenia may not be appropriate. For example, a patient who does not wish to cook may be housed close to an inexpensive cafe. It is important to assess cognitive function, since this may limit the capacity of the patient to learn and use skills [3]. If lack of function is a consequence of cognitive compromise in addition to negative symptoms, rehabilitation may prove impossible and a prosthetic environment should be supplied. Patients should not, however, be subject to overprovision that may induce further disability.

Social skills training

Negative symptoms have been found to correlate positively with deficits in social skills and inversely with total appropriate behaviour, particularly social interpersonal activity [4]. Even if this represents no more than an overlap between negative symptoms and their social manifestations, there is a possibility that social skills training may be of benefit to patients with negative symptoms simply because of the greater degree of room for improvement.

A randomized study compared a nine-week active social skills training intervention with structured activities not including social skills work [5]. The study found that both interventions were helpful in that both overall symptomatology and the need for medication were reduced. The social skills training intervention was more effective at improving negative symptoms. By six months, however, all improvements were beginning to decline, which argues for treatment to continue in some form. A small study that provided social skills training to three deficit and three non-deficit patients showed that the non-deficit patients did better than deficit patients in levels of skill acquisition and negative symptom improvements [6]. This study exemplifies the importance of assessing patients prior to such therapy in terms of their potential to benefit.

In summary, although there has been far less work on psychotherapeutic interventions aimed at negative symptoms than on pharmacological interventions, the two should be inextricably linked in the care of the individual patient. Accurate assessment of the needs and capacity to benefit of the patient is crucial and plans of therapy should be tailored specifically to these; relatives and carers should also not be excluded, as they too require an assessment of their needs and the best way to go about fulfilling them. Blanket approaches along narrow lines are unlikely to be successful. Many patients and families come to rehabilitation services with a long history of unsatisfactory treatment and disillusionment; some feel they have been blamed for the illness, while others have had years of struggling to cope before a diagnosis was made. Although it is important not to offer unrealistic promises of recovery in these circumstances, the installation of some hope is both appropriate and realistic; there are few patients for whom absolutely nothing can be done.

References

1. North CS, Pollio DE, Sachar B et al. **The family as caregiver: a group psychoeducation model for schizophrenia.** Am J Orthopsychiatry 1998; **68**:39–46.
2. Mueser KT, Valentiner DP, Agresta J. **Coping with negative symptoms of schizophrenia: patient and family prospectives.** Schizophr Bull 1997; **23**:329–339.
3. Green MF. **What are the functional consequences of neurocognitive deficits in schizophrenia?** Am J Psychiatry 1996; **153**:321–330.
4. Glynn SM, Bowen L, Rose G. **Behavioural correlates of negative symptoms in schizophrenia.** Association for Advancement of Behavior Therapy Annual Convention, San Francisco, 1990.
5. Dobson DJ, McDougall G, Busheikin J et al. **Effects of social skills training and social milieu treatment on symptoms of schizophrenia.** Psychiatr Serv 1995; **46**:376–380.
6. Kopelowicz A, Liberman RP, Mintz J et al. **Comparison of efficacy of social skills training for deficit and nondeficit negative symptoms in schizophrenia.** Am J Psychiatry 1997; **154**:424–425.

Chapter 9

Coordinating the delivery of services

Primary and secondary care

Patients with prominent negative symptoms may be even more reliant upon effective liaison between primary and secondary care than people with schizophrenia characterized by obvious positive symptoms. Whereas the latter may come to the notice of doctors and other healthcare professionals as a consequence of florid abnormalities of behaviour, the patient with pronounced negative symptoms may be hidden away, either through social withdrawal or disorganization, which may produce a spectrum of consequences, from missed appointments to homelessness.

A number of innovations in the way that mental healthcare is delivered to the community have been introduced in recent years in the UK and these will have implications for the provision of care to those most debilitated by negative symptoms. The broad range of needs that these patients have may require involvement with different members of the community mental health team (CMHT); the care of the patient may be best planned and co-ordinated through the care programming approach (CPA); and the vulnerability of the patient to deterioration may make them candidates for the supervision register. In addition, shared care protocols have emerged for the treatment of chronic disorders in the community, with general practitioners (GPs) and psychiatrists collaborating in the management of schizophrenia.

Community mental health teams

CMHTs are essentially multidisciplinary and their effective functioning calls for teamwork and ease of communication. A particular CMHT will relate to a given catchment area and should have explicit links with general practices in the vicinity. In future, such links may comprise of 'link workers', whose role it will be to liaise between primary and secondary care and to diffuse skills and knowledge in the primary care setting. Information technology may play an important part in the cohesion of such links and may greatly facilitate referrals, consultations and ensuing plans of action.

Each CMHT comprises psychiatrists (consultant and junior colleagues), community psychiatric nurses, social workers, occupational therapists and psychologists. The role of each of these members in the management of negative symptoms will now be reprised.

The psychiatrist
The psychiatrist should be available to provide diagnostic and management skills, advice on pharmacological and psychological therapies and long term surveillance, especially in those with severe and enduring mental illness. The psychiatrist is likely to be the only member of the team to prescribe for patients (although nurse practitioners

may eventually do so). In a 'seamless' service, the same consultant may manage patients who require treatment in wards, day hospitals and clinic settings. It is highly likely that the consultant psychiatrist will initiate the first prescription of an atypical antipsychotic drug (not least because of their resource implications within the UK National Heath Service). The psychiatrist should liaise with the GP about their patient and this should be reciprocated. The GP should be informed promptly when a patient is discharged home.

The community psychiatric nurse
The role of the community psychiatric nurse is changing, but with respect to patients who suffer from schizophrenia and who are resident in the community, it is likely to continue to include the monitoring of symptoms, the forming of supportive therapeutic relationships, the administration of depot neuroleptic drugs (a most reliable form of treatment in those patients who have difficulty taking tablets) and liaison with the GP. Community psychiatric nurses may provide other skills in well-resourced settings, including cognitive, behavioural and family therapies, the running of patient and carers' groups etc.

The social worker
The role of the social worker within the CMHT is also undergoing change, moving away from the provision of supportive relationships towards a care managing, co-ordinating role (eg, monitoring the provision of home support workers or appropriate accommodation). The social workers on the team will still provide information regarding benefits such as Disability Living Allowance (DLA) or travel passes. 'Approved social workers' take part in the assessment of patients being considered for detention under the UK Mental Health Act. In many areas, the approved social worker may be called upon to coordinate the 'section assessment' and will liaise with ward staff to find a psychiatric bed. The patient with negative symptoms may need to be prompted into pursuing their benefits and may need assistance in completing forms and keeping interview appointments. The patient's 'key worker' (*see* 'Care programming approach' section) may be of particular assistance in helping with these needs and will often be a social worker.

The occupational therapist
The occupational therapist has skills of particular relevance to patients with negative symptoms: assessing the performance of activities of daily living (ADL), assisting patients with training programmes aimed at enhancing self-care and motivation or rehabilitation towards sheltered work. Occupational therapists may work in the community or day hospital settings, they may run groups that focus on self-care, such as cooking and budgeting or aesthetic pursuits, such as art, pottery or sculpture.

The clinical psychologist
The clinical psychologist brings different skills to the CMHT, which may have less relevance to the treatment of those patients with severe deficit states. Patients with

pronounced negative symptoms may be unable to engage with psychological therapies, although in highly structured environments (long-stay wards and hostels) behavioural interventions may encourage self-care and limit antisocial behaviours. The clinical psychologist may, however, occasionally be called upon to perform a psychometric assessment of a patient's cognition, in order to formulate a realistic rehabilitation plan.

The relative contributions of the CMHT members may be most apparent in the management of patients subject to the CPA.

Care programming approach

The CPA was introduced in the UK in 1991. The CPA provides a model for delivering interdisciplinary care to vulnerable patients, across the health and local authorities divide, together with regular review, so that the process becomes iterative. All patients detained under the UK Mental Health Act should be subject to a CPA. Regular meetings occur, attended by all those involved in the care of the patient (including the patient) and a 'needs assessment' is performed. The needs of the patient are recorded and an action plan (or 'care plan') is devised, recorded and agreed upon by all those present at the meeting. One of the professionals involved will agree to be the patient's key worker and it is their responsibility to convene future meetings, to ensure that the patient is registered with a GP and to ensure that the care plan is acted upon. The key worker provides a constant point of contact for the patient and those involved in the care of the patient. Any unmet needs (eg, lack of suitable housing or lack of local provision of family therapy) are also recorded, and these may have an influence upon future service development. The patient's GP is invited to the CPA meetings. The key worker is usually a community psychiatric nurse or social worker, but sometimes a psychiatrist. A typical CPA care plan is outlined in Table 9.1.

Depending upon individual circumstances, voluntary agencies, relatives and carers might also have a role to play in the CPA. In the inner cities, however, many patients may live alone in hostel accommodation and those with negative symptoms may be particularly vulnerable to deterioration if statutory agencies fail to monitor their progress.

The supervision register

At the time of the CPA meeting, one decision that may have to be made is whether to place the patient on the supervision register. These registers were introduced in

Care programming approach	
Professional	**Tasks (examples)**
Community psychiatric nurse (key worker)	To monitor mental state. To administer depot depixol fortnightly. To monitor side effects
Social worker	To assist with benefits and application for hostel
Psychiatrist	To monitor mental state every two months. To consider atypical antipsychotic drug if extrapyramidal side effects continue to be problematic
General practitioner	To provide physical care (eg, if patient is a heavy smoker)
Occupational therapist	Assist in finding sheltered workshop. Review activities of daily living if swaps to an 'atypical' drug

Table 9.1. Contact details for each professional should be available.

the UK in 1994 as a way of ensuring that the most vulnerable patients seen by each CMHT were not 'lost track of' or allowed to relapse without the team being in touch with them. Those included on the register will often be patients who suffer from schizophrenia and who are considered most at risk of the following:

- Non-compliance with medication (and hence, relapse).
- Self-neglect.
- Harm to themselves.
- Harm to others.

It is clear that those with negative symptoms may be at particular risk of non-compliance and self-neglect and strenuous efforts may be required by members of the CMHT to 'keep in touch' with these patients (eg, calling at regular intervals and 'out of hours', collecting prescriptions, assisting with finances and home care and monitoring the mental state). Because of the extensive needs of these patients, they may be the focus of local initiatives such as assertive outreach nurses who have lower case numbers and more time for each client.

The general practitioner

Although GPs' experience of psychiatric illness will most often involve the management of affective disorders, neuroses, problem drinking and a variety of psychosomatic conditions, those in large practices or in inner cities are likely to have a number of patients with schizophrenia on their lists. The lifetime incidence of the condition is approximately one in 100 of the population and this is likely to be higher in urban practices. Therefore, a group practice of five or six partners may have 100–120 patients with schizophrenia. A disease register might easily be constructed by asking partners whom they see, consulting clinic and repeat prescription lists or by computer searching of prescriptions for neuroleptic drugs and other psychotropic medication. A call–recall system may assist with follow-up, especially of those who do not attend the surgery.

Preventing non-compliance with neuroleptic medication is the key to preventing relapse in schizophrenia. Hence, systematic monitoring of prescribing may prevent relapse and subsequent functional decline.

People with schizophrenia are at increased risk of cardiovascular and respiratory diseases and, thus, a screening (or 'secondary prevention') approach to managing these patients might include a system for annual review (examination by GP and/or practice nurse), with blood pressure, weight measurement, urine test and electrocardiography when indicated.

The GP may choose to see patients with schizophrenia during 'double appointments' so that there is more time to address psychological, physical and social issues. A yearly home visit by a member of the primary care team (singly or in pairs) could detect any problems such as deterioration in living conditions, unmet needs of carers etc.

Similarly, a practice audit might systematically address the following issues:

- Are the patient's personal details, including address, correct?
- Is there a key worker named in the notes?
- Are there contact numbers for the patient's key worker, community psychiatric nurse and consultant in the notes?
- Is the patient seen by anyone regularly who might detect relapse? (Is there a longstanding friend or relative who spots the 'relapse signature'? [eg, 'he starts staying up all night and not coming out of his room...'].)
- Although the patient suffers from schizophrenia, is there evidence of depression as well? (Is the patient receiving antidepressants or 'mood stabilizers' such as lithium? Mortality from suicide in schizophrenia is 10–20%. Depression may mimic the negative symptoms of schizophrenia.)
- Does the patient have side effects from their antipsychotic medication? (The motor side effects may produce secondary 'negative symptoms' [eg, apparent affective flattening with Parkinsonian facies and psychomotor retardation]. The unpleasant restlessness of akathisia may itself be associated with suicide [1–4].)
- Is there a record of drug doses and their justification? Are all neuroleptic drugs prescribed within the limits set out in the British National Formulary? (A patient who required anticholinergic medication while on 'typical'

antipsychotic drugs may not require anticholinergic medication when receiving an 'atypical' neuroleptic drug. High-dose neuroleptic medication is difficult to justify and should prompt review/discussion with the patient's consultant psychiatrist.)
- Is the treatment regimen straightforward? Might a dosset box or blister pack improve compliance?
- Is the patient on more than one neuroleptic drug? If so, why?
- Are there patient information sheets on schizophrenia and its treatment? Is there information for families? (The Royal College of Psychiatrists publishes a series of pamphlets for patients and their carers on a number of conditions, treatments, and issues to do with mental health.)
- Are there local day centres or 'drop-ins' that the patient might use? Are there support groups for the patient and their relatives?
- Financial/practical: does the patient receive any DLA? Is accommodation suitable to their needs? Are they living under sanitary conditions?
- Are all of the partners conversant with the Mental Health Act or is one experienced in its use and providing a local resource?
- Does everyone know how to initiate a Mental Health Act assessment, should the need arise?
- Are the reception staff sensitive to the special needs of the most clinically affected patients?
- Are there family members who undermine the patient, through critical remarks or over-involvement? (High 'expressed emotion' is associated with an increased risk of relapse.)

The items of information may be entered into a proforma designed to keep inside the patient's notes. Suitable practice software might also prompt the GP to update this file when the patient is reviewed.

Shared care

Shared care of many chronic diseases such as diabetes and asthma has become central to their management in the community and provides a rationale for the responsible use of clinical resources. While specialist services provide diagnostic and investigative facilities and expertise, much of the routine medical care may be provided in the context of well-resourced primary care. Detection of 'non-routine' developments leads to prompt referral, assessment and treatment in secondary care, with return to the primary care physician when the period of specialist intervention has appropriately ceased. The latter is also likely to be closer to the patient's home in the community and sustained by a longer-term relationship between the patient and the physician.

In the management of schizophrenia, it is likely that consultant psychiatrists will continue to provide expertise in the diagnosis, treatment and detailed monitoring of the mental states of affected patients, and that their teams are likely to remain involved in the provision of maintenance treatment and rehabilitative after-care. An active collaboration between the CMHT and the primary care team will, however, provide a service that is superior both in access and scope. The GP and practice nurse have a role to play in caring for the physical health of these vulnerable patients, they may also prescribe and administer maintenance treatment. By virtue of their community setting and long-term relationship they are well placed to detect changes in social conditions and the mental states of their patients. It is likely that the precise modus operandi of shared care will vary with location and other service imperatives, but effective liaison will remain central to helping the most vulnerable patients suffering from schizophrenia lead stable and fulfilling lives.

References

1. Van Putten T, Marder SR. **Behavioral toxicity of antipsychotic drugs.** *J Clin Psychiatry* 1987; **48**(Suppl. 9):13–19.
2. Ayd FJ Jr. **Akathesia and suicide: fact or myth?** *Int Drug Therapy Newslett* 1988; **23**:37–38.
3. Sachdev P. *Akathesia and Restless Legs.* Cambridge: Cambridge University Press, 1995.
4. Barnes TRE, Spence SA. **Movement disorders associated with antipsychotic drugs: clinical and biological implications.** In: *The Psychopharmacology of Schizophrenia.* Edited by MA Reveley and JFW Deakin. London: Arnold, 2000;178–210.

Source material

Barnes TR, Liddle PF, Curson DA et al. **Negative symptoms, tardive dyskinesia and depression in chronic schizophrenia.** Br J Psychiatry Suppl 1989; **155**:99–103.

Beasley CM Jr, Tollefson G, Tran P et al. **Olanzapine versus placebo and haloperidol: acute phase results of the North American double-blind olanzapine trial.** Neuropsychopharmacology 1996; **14**:111–123.

Crow TJ. **The two-syndrome concept: origins and current status.** Schizophr Bull 1985; **11**:471–486.

Hirsch SR. **Depression 'revealed' in schizophrenia.** Br J Psychiatry 1982; **140**:421–423.

Johnson DAW. **Depressive symptoms in schizophrenia: some observations on frequency, morbidity and possible causes.** In: Contemporary Issues in Schizophrenia. Edited by A Kerr and P Snaith. London: Gaskell, 1986;451–458.

Johnstone EC, Crow TJ, Frith CD. **Mechanism of the antipsychotic effect in the treatment of acute schizophrenia.** Lancet 1978; **1**:848–851.

Krawiecka M, Goldberg D, Vaughan M. **A standardized psychiatric assessment scale for rating chronic psychotic patients.** Acta Psychiatr Scand 1977; **55**:299–308.

Liddle PF. **The symptoms of chronic schizophrenia. A re-examination of the positive-negative dichotomy.** Br J Psychiatry 1987; **151**:145–151.

Lieberman JA, Fleischacker WW. **Current issues in the development of atypical antipsychotic drugs.** Br J Psychiatry 1996; **168**(Suppl. 29).

McKenna PJ. Schizophrenia and Related Syndromes. Oxford: Oxford University Press, 1994.

McKenna PJ, Lund CE, Mortimer AM. **Negative symptoms: relationship to other schizophrenic symptoms classes.** Br J Psychiatry Suppl 1989; **155**:104–107.

Mortimer AM. **New and older antipsychotics: a comparative review of appropriate use.** CNS Drugs 1994; **2**:381–396.

Mortimer AM. **The long-term treatment of schizophrenia.** Adv Psychiatr Treat 2001; (in press).

Mortimer AM, Lund CE, McKenna PJ. **The positive:negative dichotomy in schizophrenia.** Br J Psychiatry 1990; **157**:41–49.

Mortimer AM, McKenna PJ, Lund CE et al. **Rating of negative symptoms using the High Royds Evaluation of Negativity (HEN) scale.** Br J Psychiatry Suppl 1989; **155**:89–92.

Overall JE, Gorham DR. **The brief psychiatric rating scale.** Psychol Rep 1962; **10**:799–812.

Pogue-Geile MF, Harrow M. **Negative symptoms in schizophrenia: their longitudinal course and prognostic significance.** Schizophr Bull 1985; **11**:427–439.

Prosser ES, Csernansky JG, Kaplan J et al. **Depression, parkinsonian symptoms, and negative symptoms in schizophrenics treated with neuroleptics.** J Nerv Ment Dis 1987; **175**:100–105.

Wing JK, Brown GW. Institutionalism and Schizophrenia. London: Cambridge University Press, 1970.

Further reading

Andreasen NC, Roy M-A, Flaum M. **Positive and negative symptoms.** In: *Schizophrenia.* Edited by SR Hirsch and DR Weinberger. Oxford: Blackwell Science; 1995;28–45.

Burns T, Kendrick A. **Schizophrenia.** In: *Psychiatry and General Practice.* Edited by I Pullen, G Wilkinson, A Wright *et al.* London: Royal College of Psychiatrists and Royal College of General Practitioners; 1994.

Goldberg D, Gournay K. *The General Practitioner, The Psychiatrist and the Burden of Mental Health Care.* Maudsley Discussion Paper No. 1, 1997.

Leucht S, Pitschel-Walz G, Abraham D *et al.* **Efficacy and extrapyramidal side-effects of the new antipsychotics olanzapine, quetiapine, risperidone, and sertindole compared to conventional antipsychotics and placebo. A meta-analysis of randomised controlled trials.** *Schizophr Res* 1999; **35**:51–68.

McPhillips MA, Barnes TRE. **Negative symptoms.** *Curr Opin Psychiatry* 1997; **10**:30–35.

RCGP Mental Health Fellowship Schizophrenia Disease Management Pack. London: Munro and Foster Communications, 1995.

Wilkinson G, Kendrick T. *A Carer's Guide to Schizophrenia.* London: Royal Society of Medicine Press, 1996.

Appendix I:
Pre-emptive Psychosis Symptoms (PEPS)

One point each

1. The family is concerned ___
2. Excess use of alcohol ___
3. Use of street drugs (including cannabis) ___
4. Arguing with friends and family ___
5. Spending more time alone ___

Two points each

1. Sleep difficulties ___
2. Poor appetite ___
3. Depressive mood ___
4. Poor concentration ___
5. Restlessness ___
6. Tension or nervousness ___
7. Less pleasure from things ___

Three points each

1. Inability to get your mind off one or two things ___
2. Feeling of people watching you ___
3. Seeing or hearing things that others cannot ___

Five points each

1. Ideas of reference ___
2. Odd beliefs ___
3. Odd manner of thinking and speech ___
4. Inappropriate affect ___
5. Odd behaviour or appearance ___

A score of 20 points or more suggests the need for psychiatric referral.
Source: Launer M, McKean W. **The effective management of schizophrenia within primary care.** *Prog Neurol Psychiatry* 2001; in press.

Appendix II:
Brief Psychiatric Rating Scale

1. Emotional withdrawal

Deficiency in relating to the interviewer and to the interview situation. Rate only the degree to which the patient gives the impression of failing to be in emotional contact with other people during the interview.

Not present	0
Very mild: cool/reserved	1
Mild: disinterested, bored, aspontaneous	2
Moderate: answers briefly, formal, voice flat, little change in facial expression	3
Moderately severe: answers some questions only, eye contact avoided, emotional reactions absent or inappropriate	4
Severe: mute or verbal answers irrelevant, but some responses in facial expression/gestures	5
Extremely severe: no response elicited	6

2. Motor retardation

Reduction in energy level evidenced in slowed movements. Rate on the basis of observed behaviour of the patient only, do not rate on basis of patient's subjective impression of own energy level.

Not present	0
Very mild: subjective only/lack of spontaneity/slight hesitance in speech or movements	1
Mild: subjective only/lack of spontaneity/slight hesitance in speech or movements, with pauses in speech; answers brief and delayed, but in full sentences	2
Moderate: movements slowed down, speech aspontaneous, voice low, answers delayed in brief or incompatible	3
Moderately: little change in facial expression, movements slow, severely hesitant, incomplete; speech: single words, in whisper, on questions only contact; emotional reactions absent or inappropriate	4
Severe: semi-stupor	5
Extremely severe: stupor	6

3. Blunted or inappropriate affect

Reduced emotional tone, apparent lack of normal feeling or involvement. The expressed emotion is inappropriate to the situation or thought content.

Not present	0
Very mild: emotional reactions lacking in spontaneity	1
Mild: emotional reactions scarce and rigid	2
Moderate: apathetic; affect flat; little interest in family, friends, environment, own future; if delusional – delusions still affectively loaded; inappropriate grinning	3
Moderately severe: apathy and withdrawal; indifferent towards their own situation; delusions/hallucinations have no affective colouring; incongruity of affect	4
Severe: profound apathy and withdrawal; no interests; expression of affect absent or inappropriate; self-neglect in appearance and behaviour	5
Extremely severe: total apathy and indifference with self-neglect in basic needs; affect, if expressed, grossly inappropriate	6

Source: Overall JE, Gorham DR. **The brief psychiatric rating scale.** *Psychol Rep* 1962; **10**:799–812.

Appendix III: The Manchester Scale

1. Flattened incongruous affect

Flatness refers to an impairment in the range of available emotional responses; the patient is unable to convey the impact of events while relating their history and cannot convey warmth or affection while speaking about those near to them.

Absent: normal affect at interview	0
Mild: the patient may be laconic, taciturn or unresponsive in discussing emotionally charged topics, but the rater considers that this is an habitual trait rather than a sign of illness	1
Moderate: clinically significant impairment of emotional response of mild degree. Definite lack of emotional tone discussing important topics, or occasional but undoubted incongruous emotional responses during the interview	2
Marked: clinically significant impairment of emotional response of marked degree. No warmth or affection shown. Cannot convey impact of events when giving history, no concern expressed about future; or frequent incongruous responses of mild degree or occasional gross incongruity	3
Severe: clinically significant impairment of emotional response of extreme degree; no emotional response whatever elicited; or gross frequent incongruity; fatuous, supercilious, giggling, etc, in such a way as to disturb the interview	4

2. Psychomotor retardation

Absent: normal manner and speech during interview. Questions answered fairly promptly; air of spontaneity and changes of expression	0
Mild: although there may be evidence of slowness or poor spontaneity the rater considers that this is either an habitual trait or that it does not amount to clearly pathological proportions	1
Moderate: the rater detects slowness or lack of spontaneity at interview and attributes this to psychiatric illness: it is just clinically detectable. Delays in answering questions would merit this rating providing that the rater considers that it is part of a morbid mental state rather than an habitual trait of the patient	2
Marked: psychomotor retardation attributable to psychiatric illness is easily detectable at interview and is thought to make a material contribution to the abnormalities of the patient's present mental state	3
Severe: psychomotor retardation is present in extreme degree for the individual concerned	4

3. Poverty of speech, mute

Absent: speech normal in quantity and form	0
Mild: patient only speaks when spoken to; tends to give brief replies	1
Moderate: occasional difficulties or silences, but most of interview proceeds smoothly; or conversation impeded by vagueness, hesitancy or brevity of replies	2
Marked: monosyllabic replies, often long pauses or failure to answer at all; or reasonable amount of speech, but answers slow and hesitant, lacking in content, or repetitious and wandering, that meaningful conversation was almost impossible	3
Severe: mute throughout interview, or speaks only two or three words; or constantly murmuring under breath	4

Source: Krawiecka M, Goldberg D, Vaughan M. **A standardized psychiatric assessment scale for rating chronic psychotic patients.** *Acta Psychiatr Scand* 1977; **55**:299–308.
Hyde CE. **The Manchester Scale. A standardised psychiatric assessment for rating chronic psychotic patients.** *Br J Psychiatry* 1989; **155**:45–48.

Appendix IV:
The High Royds Evaluation of Negativity

? = not assessed
0 = absent
1 = questionable
2 = mild
3 = moderate
4 = severe (in general, reserved for chronically hospitalized patients)

Check one box only	?	0	1	2	3	4

1. Appearance

	?	0	1	2	3	4
Face and hair: unwashed, unshaven, hair unkempt, poor dental state (not wearing dentures = at least 2)	☐	☐	☐	☐	☐	☐
Body: dirty nails, nicotine stained fingers, body odour	☐	☐	☐	☐	☐	☐
Clothes: soiled, torn, missing buttons, holes in shoes, broken/untied shoe laces (hospital charity shop clothes = 3 or 4)	☐	☐	☐	☐	☐	☐
Global rating of appearance	☐	☐	☐	☐	☐	☐

2. Behaviour

	?	0	1	2	3	4
Reduced facial expression: rate normal animation only; disregard grimacing, dyskinesia	☐	☐	☐	☐	☐	☐
Reduced expressive gestures: rate normal gestures only; disregard stereotypes, mannerisms, dyskinesia	☐	☐	☐	☐	☐	☐
Slowness/clumsiness of movement: lack of normal ease; naturalness of movement; sits abnormally still	☐	☐	☐	☐	☐	☐
Global rating of behaviour	☐	☐	☐	☐	☐	☐

3. Speech

	?	0	1	2	3	4
Reduced in quantity: poverty of speech, distinguish from 'impoverishment of thought'	☐	☐	☐	☐	☐	☐
Lacks inflection: lacks normal modulation; monotonous; include harsh or stereotyped inflection	☐	☐	☐	☐	☐	☐
Slowness/latency of speech: measured, ponderous, laboured speech; include latency of responding	☐	☐	☐	☐	☐	☐
Global rating of speech	☐	☐	☐	☐	☐	☐

4. Thought (do not rate unless speech output adequate)

Impoverishment of thought: ideas conveyed in a repetitive, stereotyped way; keeps returning to same themes; poverty of ideation ☐ ☐ ☐ ☐ ☐ ☐

Poor performance on tests of attention/concentration: for example, months backward, serial sevens; take educational background into account ☐ ☐ ☐ ☐ ☐ ☐

Global rating of thought ☐ ☐ ☐ ☐ ☐ ☐

5. Affect

Constricted affect: reduced range of emotional expression; lack of responsiveness to social cues; indifference to emotive, eg, delusional topics ☐ ☐ ☐ ☐ ☐ ☐

Emotional withdrawnness: cold, aloof, vacant, lack of rapport ☐ ☐ ☐ ☐ ☐ ☐

Shallow/coarsened affect: emotions lack subtlety, depth of conviction; 'superficial'; 'facile'; do not rate inappropriate affect, causeless laughter etc ☐ ☐ ☐ ☐ ☐ ☐

Global rating of affect ☐ ☐ ☐ ☐ ☐ ☐

6. Functioning (past month or immediately prior to most recent admission, if acute)

Reduced interests:

    some active interests, goes out, or keeps occupied — 0/1

    more passive interests, like reading — 2

    passive television watching only — 3

    no interests, does not take in television, if watched — 4

Social withdrawal:

    actively seeks company — 0/1

    social life limited (eg, to family) — 2

    passive socialisation (eg, visits from relatives) — 3

    no interest in socialisation or relatives visits — 4

Reduced sexual interest:

    within normal limits for age, sex, circumstances — 0/1

    disproportionately diminished — 2

    minimal — 3

    total absence of interest or activity (use judgement and make allowances) — 4

Work impairment:
working regularly/part-time	0/1
working irregularly	2
unemployed or in hospital rehabilitation scheme	3
incapable of work, though may attend occupational therapist (if housekeeper, rate 0–3 on ability to perform house duties)	4

Global rating of functioning ☐ ☐ ☐ ☐ ☐ ☐

Summary score
Sum of global ratings ☐ ☐ ☐ ☐ ☐ ☐

Source: Mortimer AM, Lund CE, McKenna PJ et al. **Rating negative symptoms using the High Royds Evaluation of Negativity (HEN) scale.** Br J Psychiatry Suppl 1989; **160**:89–92.

Appendix V: Schedule for the Assessment of Negative Symptoms

1. Unchanging facial expression

Not at all: patient is normal or labile	0
Questionable decrease	1
Mild: some decrease in facial expressiveness	2
Moderate: facial expressiveness is significantly decreased	3
Marked: facial expressiveness is markedly decreased	4
Severe: facial expressiveness is essentially unchanging	5

2. Decreased spontaneous movements

Not at all: patient moves normally or is overactive	0
Questionable decrease	1
Mild: some decrease in spontaneous movements	2
Moderate: significant decrease in spontaneous movements	3
Marked: movements are markedly decreased	4
Severe: patient sits immobile throughout the interview	5

3. Paucity of expressive gestures

Not at all: patient uses expressive gestures normally or excessively	0
Questionable decrease	1
Mild: some decrease in expressive gestures	2
Moderate: significant decrease in expressive gestures	3
Marked: marked decrease in gestures	4
Severe: patient never used body as an aid in expression	5

4. Poor eye contact

Not at all: good eye contact and expression	0
Questionable decrease	1
Mild: some decrease in eye contact and expression	2
Moderate: significant decrease eye contact and expression	3

Marked: very infrequent eye contact	4
Severe: patient almost never looks at interviewer	5

5. Affective nonresponsivity

Not at all	0
Questionable decrease	1
Mild: slight but definite lack of responsivity	2
Moderate: moderate decrease in responsivity	3
Marked: marked decrease in responsivity	4
Severe: patient essentially unresponsive, even on prompting	5

6. Inappropriate affect

Not at all: affect is not appropriate	0
Questionable	1
Mild: at least one instance of inappropriate smiling or other inappropriate affect	2
Moderate: occasional instances of inappropriate affect	3
Marked: frequent instances of inappropriate affect	4
Severe: affect is inappropriate most of the time	5

7. Lack of vocal inflections

Not at all: normal vocal inflections	0
Questionable decrease	1
Mild: slight decrease in vocal inflections	2
Moderate: definite decrease in vocal inflections	3
Marked: marked decrease in vocal inflections	4
Severe: nearly all speech seems to be in a monotone	5

8. Subjective complaints of emotional emptiness or loss of feeling

Not at all: patient reports normal intensity of affect or increased intensity	0
Questionable	1
Mild: slight but definite decrease in subjective feelings	2
Moderate: moderate decrease in feeling	3
Marked: significant decrease in feeling	4

Severe: the patient describes themselves as unable to feel normally most of the time   5

9. Global rating of affective flattening

No flattening: normal affect	0
Questionable affective flattening	1
Mild affective flattening	2
Moderate affective flattening	3
Marked affective flattening	4
Severe affective flattening	5

10. Poverty of speech

No poverty of speech: a substantial and appropriate number of replies to questions including additional information	0
Questionable poverty of speech	1
Slight poverty of speech: occasional replies do not include elaborated information even though this is appropriate	2
Moderate poverty of speech: some replies do not include appropriately elaborated information and many replies are monosyllabic or very brief ('yes', 'no', 'maybe', 'don't know', 'last week')	3
Marked poverty of speech: answers are rarely more than a few words in length	4
Severe poverty of speech: patient says very little and occasionally fails to answer questions	5

11. Poverty of content of speech

No poverty of content of speech	0
Questionable poverty of content of speech	1
Mild poverty of content of speech: occasional replies are too vague to be comprehensible or can be markedly condensed	2
Moderate poverty of content of speech: frequent replies which are vague or can be markedly condensed to make up at least a quarter of the interview	3
Marked poverty of content of speech: at least half of the patient's speech is composed of vague or incomprehensible replies	4
Severe poverty of content of speech: nearly all the patient's speech is vague, incomprehensible, or can be markedly condensed	5

12. Blocking

No blocking	0
Questionable blocking	1
Mild blocking: a single instance noted during a 15-minute period	2
Moderate blocking: occurs twice during 15 minutes	3
Marked blocking: occurs three times during 15 minutes	4
Severe blocking: occurs more than three times	5

13. Increased latency of response

Not at all: patient typically replies promptly	0
Questionable	1
Mild: occasional brief pause before replying	2
Moderate: significant decrease in latency of response	3
Marked: marked decrease in latency of response	4
Severe: long pauses prior to nearly all replies	5

14. Subjective rating of alogia

Not at all: no subjective complaints of empty thoughts	0
Questionable	1
Mild: the patient reports some slight but definite decrease	2
Moderate: the patient notes a significant decrease	3
Marked: the patient reports a substantial decrease	4
Severe: the patient reports that much of the time their mind seems empty and that they have difficulty in developing their thoughts	5

15. Global rating of alogia

No alogia	0
Questionable alogia	1
Mild: mild, but definite impoverishment in thinking	2
Moderate: significant evidence for impoverished thinking	3
Marked: patient's thinking seems impoverished much of the time	4
Severe: patient's thinking seems impoverished nearly all of the time	5

16. Grooming and hygiene

No evidence of poor grooming and hygiene	0
Questionable impairment	1
Mild: some slight, but definite indication of inattention to appearance	2
Moderate: appearance is somewhat dishevelled	3
Marked: appearance is significantly dishevelled	4
Severe: appearance is severely dishevelled	5

17. Impersistence at work or school

No evidence of impersistence at work or school	0
Questionable	1
Mild: slight indications of impersistence	2
Moderate: definite indications of impersistence	3
Marked: significant indications of impersistence	4
Severe: patient has consistently failed to maintain a work record or attend school	5

18. Physical anergia

No evidence of physical anergia	0
Questionable	1
Mild anergia	2
Moderate anergia	3
Marked anergia	4
Severe anergia	5

19. Subjective complaints of avolition and apathy

No complaints	0
Questionable	1
Mild but definite complaints	2
Moderate complaints	3
Marked complaints	4
Severe complaints	5

20. Global rating of avolition and apathy

No avolition	0
Questionable	1
Mild but definitely present	2
Moderate avolition	3
Marked avolition	4
Severe avolition	5

21. Recreational interests and activities

No inability to enjoy recreational activities	0
Questionable	1
Mild inability to enjoy recreational activities	2
Moderate inability to enjoy recreational activities	3
Marked inability to enjoy recreational activities	4
Severe inability to enjoy recreational activities	5

22. Sexual interest and activity

No inability to enjoy sexual activities	0
Questionable loss of ability to enjoy sex	1
Mild but definite loss of ability to enjoy sex	2
Moderate loss of ability to enjoy sex	3
Marked loss of ability to enjoy sex	4
Severe loss of ability to enjoy sex	5

23. Ability to feel intimacy and closeness

No inability to feel intimacy and closeness	0
Questionable inability	1
Mild but definite inability to feel intimacy and closeness	2
Moderate inability to feel intimacy and closeness	3
Marked inability to feel intimacy and closeness	4
Severe inability to feel intimacy and closeness	5

24. Relationships with friends and peers

No inability to form friendships	0
Questionable inability to form friendships	1
Mild inability to form friendships	2
Moderate inability to form friendships	3
Marked inability to form friendships	4
Severe inability to form friendships	5

25. Subjective awareness of anhedonia-associality

No subjective awareness of anhedonia-associality	0
Questionable awareness of anhedonia-associality	1
Mild but definite awareness of anhedonia-associality	2
Moderate awareness of anhedonia-associality	3
Marked awareness of anhedonia-associality	4
Severe awareness of anhedonia-associality	5

26. Global rating of anhedonia-associality

No evidence of anhedonia-associality	0
Questionable evidence of anhedonia-associality	1
Mild but definite evidence of anhedonia-associality	2
Moderate evidence of anhedonia-associality	3
Marked evidence of anhedonia-associality	4
Severe evidence of anhedonia-associality	5

27. Social inattentiveness

No indication of inattentiveness	0
Questionable signs of inattentiveness	1
Mild but definite signs of inattentiveness	2
Moderate signs of inattentiveness	3
Marked signs of inattentiveness	4
Severe signs of inattentiveness	5

28. Inattentiveness during mental status testing

No errors	0
Questionable: no errors, but the patient performs in a halting manner or makes an error and corrects it	1
Mild but definite: one error	2
Moderate: two errors	3
Marked: three errors	4
Severe: more than three errors	5

29. Subjective complaints of inattentiveness

No complaints	0
Questionable	1
Mild but definite complaints	2
Moderate complaints	3
Marked complaints	4
Severe complaints	5

30. Global rating of inattentiveness

No indications of inattentiveness	0
Questionable	1
Mild but definite inattentiveness	2
Moderate inattentiveness	3
Marked inattentiveness	4
Severe inattentiveness	5

Source: Andreasen NC. *The Comprehensive Assessment of Symptoms and History.* Iowa City: The University of Iowa College of Medicine, 1987.

Appendix VI:
The Positive and Negative Syndromes of Schizophrenia (Negative subscale)

1. Blunted affect

Diminished emotional responsiveness as characterized by a reduction in facial expression, modulation of feelings and communicative gestures. Basis for rating: observation of physical manifestations of affective tone and emotional responsiveness during the course of the interview.

Absent: definition does not apply	1
Minimal: questionable pathology; may be at the upper extreme of normal limits	2
Mild: changes in facial expression and communicative gestures seem to be stilted, forced, artificial, or lacking in modulation	3
Moderate: reduced range of facial expression and few expressive gestures result in dull appearance	4
Moderate severe: affect is generally 'flat' with only occasional changes in facial expression; paucity of communicative gestures	5
Severe: marked flatness and deficiency of emotions exhibited most of the time. There may be unmodulated extreme affective discharges, such as excitement, rage, or inappropriate uncontrolled laughter	6
Extreme: changes in facial expression and evidence of communicative gestures are virtually absent. Patient seems constantly to show a barren or 'wooden' expression	7

2. Emotional withdrawal

Lack of interest in, involvement with, and affective commitment to life's events. Basis for rating: reports of functioning from primary care workers or family and observation of interpersonal behaviour during the course of the interview.

Absent: definition does not apply	1
Minimal: questionable pathology; may be at the upper extreme of normal limits	2
Mild: usually lacks initiative and occasionally may show deficient interest in surrounding events	3
Moderate: patient is generally distanced emotionally from the milieu and its challenges, but, with encouragement, can be engaged	4
Moderate severe: patient is clearly detached emotionally from persons and events in the milieu, resisting all efforts at engagement. Patient appears distant, docile and purposeless, but can be involved in communication at least briefly and tends to personal needs, sometimes with assistance	5

Severe: marked deficiency of interest and emotional commitment results in limited conversation with others and frequent neglect of personal functions, for which the patient requires supervision	6
Extreme: patient is almost totally withdrawn, uncommunicative, and neglectful of personal needs as a result of profound lack of interest and emotional commitment	7

3. Poor rapport

Lack of interpersonal empathy, openness in conversation and sense of closeness, interest or involvement with the interviewer. This is evidenced by interpersonal distancing and reduced verbal and nonverbal communication. Basis for rating: interpersonal behaviour during the course of the interview.

Absent: definition does not apply	1
Minimal: questionable pathology; may be at the upper extreme of normal limits	2
Mild: conversation is characterized by a stilted, strained, or artificial tone. It may lack emotional depth or tend to remain on an impersonal, intellectual plane	3
Moderate: patient typically is aloof, with interpersonal distance quite evident. Patient may answer questions mechanically, act bored, or express disinterest	4
Moderate severe: disinvolvement is obvious and clearly impedes the productivity of the interview. Patient may tend to avoid eye or face contact	5
Severe: patient is highly indifferent, with marked interpersonal distance. Answers are perfunctory and there is little nonverbal evidence of involvement. Eye and face contact are frequently avoided	6
Extreme: patient is totally uninvolved with the interviewer. Patient appears to be completely indifferent and consistently avoids verbal and nonverbal interactions during the interview	7

4. Passive/apathetic social withdrawal

Diminished interest and initiative in social interactions due to passivity, apathy, anergy or avolition. This leads to reduced interpersonal involvement and neglect of activities of daily living. Basis for rating: reports on social behaviour from primary care workers or family.

Absent: definition does not apply	1
Minimal: questionable pathology; may be at the upper extreme of normal limits	2
Mild: shows occasional interest in social activities but poor initiative. Usually engages with others only when approached first by them	3
Moderate: passively goes along with most social activities but in a disinterested or mechanical way. Tends to recede into the background	4
Moderate severe: passively participates in only a minority of activities and shows virtually no interest or initiative. Generally spends little time with others	5

Severe: tends to be apathetic and isolated, participating very rarely in social activities and occasionally neglecting personal needs. Has very few spontaneous social contacts — 6

Extreme: profoundly apathetic, socially isolated and personally neglectful — 7

5. Difficulty in abstract thinking

Impairment in the use of the abstract-symbolic mode of thinking, as evidenced by difficulty in classification, forming generalizations and proceeding beyond concrete or egocentric thinking in problem solving tasks. Basis for rating: responses to questions on similarities and proverb interpretation, and use of concrete versus abstract mode during the course of the interview.

Absent: definition does not apply — 1

Minimal: questionable pathology; may be at the upper extreme of normal limits — 2

Mild: tends to give literal or personalized interpretations to the more difficult proverbs and may have some problems with concepts that are fairly abstract or remotely related — 3

Moderate: often utilizes a concrete mode. Has difficulty with most proverbs and some categories. Tends to be distracted by functional aspects and salient features — 4

Moderate severe: deals primarily in a concrete mode, exhibiting difficulty with most proverbs and many categories — 5

Severe: unable to grasp the abstract meaning of any proverbs or figurative expressions and can formulate classifications for only the most simple of similarities. Thinking is either vacuous or locked into functional aspects, salient features and idiosyncratic interpretations — 6

Extreme: can use only concrete modes of thinking. Shows no comprehension of proverbs, common metaphors or similes, and simple categories. Even salient and functional attributes do not serve as a basis for classification. This rating may apply to those who cannot interact even minimally with the examiner because of marked cognitive impairment — 7

6. Lack of spontaneity and flow of conversation

Reduction in the normal flow of communication associated with apathy, avolition, defensiveness, or cognitive deficit. This is manifested by diminished fluidity and productivity of the verbal-interactional process. Basis for rating: cognitive-verbal processes observed during the course of the interview.

Absent: definition does not apply — 1

Minimal: questionable pathology; may be at the upper extreme of normal limits — 2

Mild: conversation shows little initiative. Patient's answers tend to be brief and unembellished, requiring direct and leading questions by the interviewer — 3

Moderate: conversation lacks free flow and appears uneven or halting. Leading — 4 questions are frequently needed to elicit adequate responses and proceed with conversation

Moderate severe: patient shows a marked lack of spontaneity and openness, replying to the interviewer's questions with only one or two brief sentences — 5

Severe: patient's responses are limited mainly to a few words or short phrases intended to avoid or curtail communication. (eg, 'I don't know', 'I'm not at liberty to say'.) Conversation is seriously impaired as a result, and the interview is highly unproductive — 6

Extreme: verbal output is restricted to, at most, an occasional utterance, making conversation not possible — 7

7. Stereotyped thinking

Decreased fluidity, spontaneity and flexibility of thinking, as evidenced in rigid, repetitious or barren thought content. Basis for rating: cognitive-verbal processes observed during the interview.

Absent: definition does not apply — 1

Minimal: questionable pathology; may be at the upper extreme of normal limits — 2

Mild: some rigidity shown in attitudes or beliefs. Patient may refuse to consider alternative positions or have difficulty in shifting from one idea to another — 3

Moderate: conversation revolves around a recurrent theme, resulting in difficulty in shifting to a new topic — 4

Moderate severe: thinking is rigid and repetitious to the point that, despite the interviewer's efforts, conversation is limited to only two or three dominating topics — 5

Severe: uncontrolled repetition of demands, statements, ideas, or questions that severely impairs conversation — 6

Extreme: thinking, behaviour and conversation are dominated by constant repetition of fixed ideas or limited phrases, leading to gross rigidity, inappropriateness and restrictiveness of the patient's communication — 7

Source: Kay SR, Opler LA, Lindenmayer JP. **The Positive and Negative Syndrome Scale (PANSS): rationale and standardisation.** *Br J Psychiatry Suppl* 1989; **155**:59–67.

Appendix VII

National Schizophrenia Fellowship
25a Outram Street
Sutton in Ashfield
Nottingham
NG17 4BA
Tel: 01623 551338
http://www.nsf.org.uk

Mind
Granta House
15–19 The Broadway
London
E15 4BQ
Tel: 020 8519 2122
http://www.mind.org.uk

SANE
1st Floor
Cityside House
40 Adler Street
London
E1 1EE
Tel: 020 7375 1002
http://www.sane.org.uk

Making Space
46 Allen Street
Warrington
Cheshire
WA2 7JB
Tel: 01925 571680
http://ds.dialpipex.com/comcare/making-space